DR. KOUFMAN'S ACID REFLUX DIET

Also by Dr. Jamie Koufman

Dropping Acid: The Reflux Diet Cookbook & Cure

The Chronic Cough Enigma

Acid Reflux in Children

DR. KOUFMAN'S ACID REFLUX DIET

111 All New Reflux-Friendly Recipes
Including Vegan & Gluten-Free

Dr. Jamie Koufman
Sonia Huang & Chef Philip Gelb

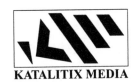

KATALITIX MEDIA

NOTICE AND DISCLAIMER

This book is intended as a reference volume only, not as a medical manual. The information given here is designed to help you make informed decisions about your health. It is not intended as a substitute for any treatment that might have been pre-scribed by your doctor. If you suspect that you have a medical problem, we urge you to seek medical help. Any use of this book is at the reader's discretion, as the advice and strategies contained within may not be suitable for every individual.

In this book, recipes and ingredients are designated as *Gluten-Free* (GF), *May-or-May-not-be-Gluten-Free* (MMGF), *Not Gluten-Free* (NGF), *Dairy-Free* (DF), and/or *Possible Trigger* food (PT). The specific GF and DF designations of ingredi-ents are shown on pages 228–234. Some ingredients are designated as NGF (not gluten-free), but we have not rated every possible NGF item. The designation MMGF is usually brand-dependant, that is, some brands are GF and some are not.

You as the consumer must carefully read product labels. If you are gluten-sensitive and in doubt, look for "GF" on the product packaging. Unless a product is specif-ically labeled as GF, there may be cross-contamination; and therefore, if you are GF or DF for medical reasons, you must be personally responsible for checking all of your own ingredients, including all of those used in the recipes and recom-mended in this book. Foods that we recognize to be reflux trigger foods are designated as PT (Possible Trigger food); however, any food can be a trigger food for any individual, and we do not take responsibility for the possibility that some of our recipes may contain ingredients that contain one or more of any individual's specific trigger food(s).

Mention of specific companies, organizations, or authorities in this book does not imply endorsement by the authors or the publisher, nor does mention of specific companies, organizations, or authorities imply that they endorse this book.

Cover by Charles Kreloff

For additional information, see: www.JamieKoufman.com
and www.KoufmanConsulting.com

For Marsha

CONTENTS

COOKING FOR LONGEVITY

RECIPES

FOREWORD

When I first met Dr. Jamie Koufman I was having a tough time, and by tough, I mean I felt like I was dying. I was waking up in the middle of the night gasping for air as my throat and vocal cords went into spasms caused by acid reflux. It was terrifying. I had had reflux before, but this was much worse than anything I had experienced.

I had seen ear, nose, and throat doctors, but they did not link my reflux to my other symptoms such as constant throat clearing, postnasal drip, and excessive morning throat phlegm. My voice was often hoarse, and my vocal cords looked like inflamed, frayed ropes—a significant professional disability for a television reporter. No doctor ever told me that the granulomas (growths) on my vocal cords were caused by reflux, too.

Dr. Koufman became my voice and reflux doctor, and she explained how my symptoms were all related to reflux. Thanks to her, I understand reflux and my voice is fine now.

Dr. Koufman taught me a lot about respiratory reflux. I read her journal articles and listened as she explained about the different stages of reflux and about the many different conditions that are caused by acid reflux. Dr. Koufman is way ahead of her time—the medical mainstream still does not understand that reflux is much more than just heartburn and indigestion. So, Dr. Koufman's new term, *respiratory reflux*, encompasses the myriad aspects of acid reflux that affect the respiratory tract.

As medical professionals and the public begin to understand the full range of respiratory reflux, the question will become: So what do I do now, especially if I don't want to take acid-blocking drugs forever?

Dr. Koufman's Acid Reflux Diet is the answer. The recipes that Dr. Koufman, Sonia Huang, and Chef Philip Gelb have created are not just tasty, they will also help you conquer your acid reflux and ease your respiratory symptoms, and, as an added bonus, they are heart healthy, too. I know because I've tried them.

I have been telling viewers about acid reflux, including respiratory reflux, ever since I became Dr. Koufman's patient. Millions of Americans are taking medications they don't need and suffering from symptoms they shouldn't have. Indeed, as Dr. Koufman puts it, the fix is a healthy diet and lifestyle that is lean, clean, green, and alkaline.

It's all here in *Dr. Koufman's Acid Reflux Diet*. Try this diet. You will enjoy it—and you'll feel better too!

Dr. Max Gomez, Medical Correspondent CBS TV

Dr. Koufman's Acid Reflux Diet

PREFACE

When Mother Cooked–Redux

Born in 1947, I am a prime-time Baby Boomer, and the world has dramatically changed in my lifetime. There were two billion people on the planet in 1950, and now there are over seven billion. As the population has grown, so too has the food industry. Much of the food we eat today is not the same as it was just 50 years ago, and the changes have resulted in widespread, often life-threatening diseases such as obesity, diabetes, asthma, heart disease, and acid reflux.[1-5]

When I was a child, my mother had dinner on the table promptly at 6 o'clock every night. Once a month we went out to eat at a steakhouse or a Chinese restaurant. All the food we consumed was local. We actually knew the man who supplied our chickens, and we got corn on the cob in late July or August when it ripened on the farm two miles from our house.

In those days, there was no such thing as fast food, no soda machines, and no Food and Drug Administration (FDA)–approved list of "Generally Recognized as Safe" (GRAS) food additives.[1,6-8] Wouldn't it be nice if we could go back to that earlier time and eat the way we did before food changed so much for the worse?

I have spent my career as a physician and scientist focused on the problem of acid reflux. With the 2010 publication of *Dropping Acid: The Reflux Diet Cookbook & Cure*,[1] the floodgates opened in my practice—I suspect because of the three words *reflux, diet,* and *cure*. That book is still the most popular book on acid reflux. Since its publication, I have continued to learn about healthy eating, and almost everything that I know about reflux and nutrition I have learned from my reflux patients.

Dropping Acid: The Reflux Diet Cookbook & Cure will help you conquer reflux through healthy diet and lifestyle. But if that book has one flaw, it is that it assumes the maintenance phase is intuitive: just avoid trigger foods and eat healthy. *Dr. Koufman's Acid Reflux Diet* is its companion book designed for the long haul. This is intended to be a longevity diet that is demanding and assumes that you are willing to make changes in what you eat and when you eat it.

When Sonia Huang, my outstanding physician assistant, suggested that we write a cookbook, I seized the opportunity. As Sonia and I worked with reflux patients individually to establish dietary health, we often observed a transformation that included weight loss and collateral disease control. In many cases, patients were able to come off their cholesterol and diabetes medications.

Sonia was the stimulus for our collaboration with her friend Chef Philip. I wrote the medical and dietary sections of this book, and Sonia and Chef Philip developed a range of delicious new recipes, most of which are vegan and gluten-free. Together, in this book we offer a new and healthier approach to eating.

Jamie Koufman, New York, October 2015

WHAT YOU
EAT IS
EATING YOU

CHAPTER 1

How Do I Know if I Have Reflux?

I n 1987, I developed the Reflux Symptom Index (RSI), and it has stood the test of time as a reliable clinical tool.[9-11] Today, it is used by physicians around the world.

Before turning the page, take the RSI quiz below and add up your score. Many people have "silent acid reflux" and don't know it. See if you do.

THE REFLUX SYMPTOM INDEX (RSI)
How do the following affect you? 0 = No Problem   5 = Severe Problem

Hoarseness or a problem with your voice	0	1	2	3	4	5
Clearing your throat	0	1	2	3	4	5
Excess throat mucous or postnasal drip	0	1	2	3	4	5
Difficulty swallowing food, liquids, pills	0	1	2	3	4	5
Coughing after you ate or lying down	0	1	2	3	4	5
Breathing difficulty or choking episodes	0	1	2	3	4	5
Troublesome or annoying cough	0	1	2	3	4	5
Sensations of a lump in your throat	0	1	2	3	4	5
Heartburn, chest pain, or indigestion	0	1	2	3	4	5

There is no one number that proves you have reflux. You can have reflux even if your score is low. If your score is 15 or greater, you have a 90 percent chance of having reflux.[1]

RSI

CHAPTER 2

Reflux and Longevity

S ince the 1960s, artificial food, hazardous chemicals, trans fats, high-fructose corn syrup, hybridized and genetically modified foods, toxic preservatives and other additives have caused the most prevalent and preventable diseases of our time. The unhealthy American diet is responsible for epidemics of obesity, diabetes, heart disease, osteoporosis, asthma, sleep apnea, acid reflux, and esophageal cancer.[1-5,8]

> **Reflux-related diseases affect at least half of Americans. Since the 1970s, the prevalence of reflux disease has increased 400 percent, and reflux-caused esophageal cancer has increased more than 850 percent; in terms of incidence, it has become America's fastest growing cancer.[8]**

In just 40 years, the acid reflux epidemic has occurred despite more than $1.5 trillion spent on medical surveillance procedures, such as endoscopy, and widespread use of acid-suppressive medications, the most notable being proton pump inhibitors (PPIs). Although they seldom control reflux, we spend $15 billion a year on PPIs alone.

The impact of the Western diet is now global, and where the Western diet goes, a reflux epidemic follows. Interestingly, the rise in reflux disease directly parallels the arc of soft drink consumption. However, while the relationship between sugary soft drinks and obesity and diabetes is in the news, another negative impact of soft drinks on our health is being ignored.

Acids—most commonly citric, phosphoric, and ascorbic, often just labeled as *vitamin C*—are the main preservatives in almost everything in a bottle or can.[1] Today, fruit juices, vitamin waters, energy drinks, and soft drinks all have the same acidity as stomach acid, and this causes serious problems for people with reflux. In fact, these products are the actual *cause* of reflux for many people.

Mandated by the FDA in 1973 following an outbreak of food poisoning, acid became the main preservative in almost every bottled and canned beverage.[1] While excessive dietary acid plays a major role in reflux disease, it may also be a factor in osteoporosis and osteopenia (bone loss) in women and prostate health in men, and it may even play a role in cancer prognosis.

Thankfully, there is good news. We can take control of our lives and restore our health. By acting responsibly and addressing dietary and lifestyle issues, we can not only beat acid reflux but reverse other serious diseases such as obesity, asthma, sleep apnea, and diabetes.

This book is about how my patients have successfully done just that. It is about weight loss, health maintenance, and disease prevention. *Dr. Koufman's Acid Reflux Diet* is the never-need-to-diet-again diet.

For 35 years, reflux, particularly respiratory reflux—acid reflux that affects the nose, sinuses, throat, vocal cords, trachea, bronchi, and lungs—has been the focus of my work as a practicing physician, scientist, and researcher.[1, 8-32] Throughout that time, I have been troubled by mainstream medicine's failure to understand reflux disease, and particularly the notion that pills and surgical procedures are the answer.

Physicians don't always recognize that personal responsibility is a patient's option. The belief, shared by doctors and patients, appears to be that patients are noncompliant and unwilling to change. Just give me a pill, demands the patient, or better yet, a surgical procedure to end my reflux. But patients need help understanding that unhealthy lifestyles cause disease and that change is possible.

The emphasis of *Dropping Acid: The Reflux Diet Cookbook & Cure* is the reflux detox, the induction phase of the reflux diet, which allows most people to gain control of reflux disease. The detox phase is both strict and restrictive, a two-week diet that is intended to make a big difference.[1,8] I may have mistakenly assumed that the maintenance phase was obvious—just eat a healthy diet—but how to define *healthy* has changed.

In recent years, a consumer-led revolt against the food industry has resulted in the banning of trans fats, the removal of genetically modified foods and artificial chemicals from many fast foods and breakfast cereals, and a notable national decrease in soft drink consumption. We now know a lot more about the harmful effects of chemicals in food, hybridized wheat, and sugar addiction, as well as the differences between "good" and "bad" fats. And as of this writing, for example, 30 percent of Americans claim to be gluten-free.

In the years since the publication of *Dropping Acid: The Reflux Diet Cookbook & Cure*, Sonia and I have worked with thousands of patients to create long-term and customized dietary and lifestyle programs. Many patients following these programs stop needing medications for high cholesterol, and their diabetes and overall health is restored. Weight loss comes naturally, too. Many patients leave our care weighing what they did in high school.

For obese patients, I may further restrict the diet—gluten-free, sugar-free, and dairy-free—with the goal of accelerating weight loss through ultra-clean eating. For more about this, see Pick Your Poison or Cure (page 75) in "The Longevity Diet" chapter.

Dr. Koufman's Acid Reflux Diet offers the reader what we have learned about dietary health since 2010, and it presents a blueprint for the long haul. This diet is not a fad, and there is no one right way to follow it. We recognize that people are different and must make individual choices.

This book advocates a diet that is *lean* (not too much red meat, milk, and other unhealthy fats), *clean* (avoidance of unpronounceable and potentially harmful chemicals), *green* (organic), and *alkaline* (low acid and pH balanced, limiting consumption of acidic foods and beverages). We also advocate portion control and consuming the equivalent of five meals a day—breakfast, snack, lunch, snack, and dinner—with dinner being a light meal eaten relatively early in the evening. We believe that we have created a paradigm shift in healthy eating.

I live in New York City with millions of foodies. So, what's the paradigm shift? Imagine this: You are invited to a dinner party at 8:30 on a Saturday night. From 8:30 to 9:30, you have hors d'oeuvres and a glass of wine. Then, you sit down to two or three courses of rich food plus a chocolate dessert. During dinner, you and your fellow diners consume two additional bottles of wine, and you push back from the table at midnight. Perhaps you have an after-dinner digestif, and you're at home and in bed around 1:00 a.m.

It would not surprise me to learn that most, if not all, of the people at that dinner party have potentially life-threatening reflux-related diseases. One might have asthma or chronic obstructive pulmonary disease (COPD), one might have snoring and sleep apnea, one might have had multiple sinus surgeries. And the worst possibility? A few years later, one of the guests gets esophageal cancer and dies at a young age. Everyone is surprised because he had no apparent symptoms, and it seemed to come without warning.

Subconsciously, many people recognize that their diseases are related to their diet and lifestyle, but they are unwilling to make the necessary changes. This is called denial. Indeed, millions of Americans are in denial, but in this book, we call out the necessary changes loudly and with conviction.

We are already in the middle of a health revolution that is food- and nutrition-related.[5] The current rejection of unhealthy food and unhealthy eating will eventually force every American to take stock of her or his diet and lifestyle.

Dr. Koufman's Acid Reflux Diet is an opportunity to start over. Yes, it does require that you always think about what, how, and when you eat. If you take our advice, you will be planning your meals for the week ahead and cooking more of your own food.

Healthy eating requires work, but it is the best road to functional longevity. This book offers an eating reboot that for many people will not be easy. Thankfully, Sonia and Chef Philip have contributed great recipes so that healthy eating can also be delicious.

Now more than ever, you are what you eat.

CHAPTER 3

The Reflux Conundrum

A cid reflux is the most prevalent and misunderstood disease of our time. It is so pervasive that it is almost invisible. For patients and doctors alike, reflux is a confusing and difficult problem.

This chapter provides background and context for this book, and it is intentionally abbreviated. If you are interested in the science and research, please read *Dropping Acid: The Reflux Diet Cookbook & Cure*,[1] particularly the front matter and the chapter "Reflux Science You Can Digest."

Respiratory Reflux: The Missing Link

The word *reflux* literally means "backflow." It is the backflow of the gastric (stomach) contents into both the esophagus—the swallowing tube that goes from the throat to the stomach—and the throat. Reflux into the esophagus is called *gastroesophageal reflux*. If it damages the esophagus or causes symptoms, then it is called *gastroesophageal reflux disease,* or GERD. *Esophageal reflux* is a simpler term, and throughout this book it will be used in place of GERD.

When gastric reflux escapes from the esophagus upward into the throat and respiratory tract, it is usually called *laryngopharyngeal reflux,* or LPR, and sometimes *airway reflux* or *silent reflux.* All of these medical terms are mine, but in this book I am introducing a new term, *respiratory reflux*, which is both descriptive and intuitive, and will be used instead of LPR.

Respiratory reflux includes reflux into the nose, sinuses, throat, voice box, trachea, bronchial tubes, and lungs. Respiratory reflux causes, or complicates, almost all respiratory diseases, including many that are still not recognized as reflux-related. In fact, respiratory reflux is a main cause of sinus disease, sleep apnea, and cancer of the esophagus, throat, and lungs.

Respiratory reflux affects millions of people who do not have digestive symptoms, so they and their doctors are unaware of the problem.

> In my experience, the three most common misdiagnoses in America are allergies, sinus disease, and asthma, with as many as three-quarters of the cases actually being caused by respiratory reflux.

Reflux Is Not About Heartburn

You do not have to have heartburn to have reflux. In fact, respiratory reflux symptoms—postnasal drip, chronic throat clearing and cough, sore throat, hoarseness, lump-in-the-throat sensation, difficulty swallowing—are far more common than heartburn, the primary symptom of esophageal reflux. This misconception among patients and physicians—that heartburn is acid reflux—has had colossal negative health consequences.

I recently examined data from my reflux patients using the Reflux Symptom Index (the quiz provided on page 3). Here were the symptoms, in decreasing order of frequency:

1. Too much throat mucus
2. Chronic throat clearing
3. Hoarseness
4. Lump-in-the throat sensation
5. Chronic cough
6. Heartburn
7. Difficulty swallowing
8. Choking episodes

Not only was heartburn only the sixth-most common symptom, heartburn was the chief complaint or primary symptom of only seven percent of the patients. Furthermore, almost half said that they had never had heartburn! Look at these results from the one-question poll on the www.refluxcookbookblog.com website:

Think you might have reflux? Which symptoms do you have?

1. Post-nasal drip	15%
2. Chronic throat-clearing	14%
3. Lump-in-the-throat sensation	14%
4. Hoarseness	12%
5. Sore throat	11%
6. Heartburn	10%
7. Chronic cough	9%
8. Difficulty swallowing	8%
9. Choking episodes	7%

With over 55,000 respondents, the results confirm that reflux is not just about heartburn. The data also suggest that most people have multiple symptoms of respiratory reflux. Indeed, most respiratory reflux patients have an average of six of the above symptoms. That is an important clinical observation: many symptoms suggest respiratory reflux and not another diagnosis.

If the above findings represent the population at large, and there is no reason to think otherwise, poorly recognized respiratory reflux is a much bigger and more important problem than esophageal reflux. Symptoms like postnasal drip, too much throat mucus, and chronic throat clearing are the tip of a massive respiratory reflux iceberg that affects almost 20 percent of the population, or over 60 million people.[8]

Manifestations of Reflux

Would it surprise you to know that respiratory reflux can cause any respiratory symptom or disease? It can even cause life-threatening lung diseases, not just common problems like postnasal drip. Listed on the next page are many of the symptoms and conditions that are reflux-related.

REFLUX-RELATED SYMPTOMS AND CONDITIONS†
Respiratory Reflux and Esophageal Reflux

SYMPTOMS	CONDITIONS
Heartburn	Esophagitis
Regurgitation	Dental and gum disease
Chest pain	Esophageal spasm
Shortness of breath	Esophageal stricture
Choking episodes	Esophageal cancer
Hoarseness	Reflux laryngitis
Vocal fatigue	Laryngeal and vocal cord cancer
Voice breaks	Endotracheal intubation injury
Chronic throat clearing	Contact ulcers and granulomas
Excessive throat mucus	Subglottic stenosis
Postnasal drip	Arytenoid fixation
Chronic cough	Paroxysmal laryngospasm
Dysphagia	Globus pharyngeus
Difficulty swallowing	Throat cancer
Difficulty breathing	Vocal cord dysfunction
Wheezing	Paradoxical vocal cord movement
Globus	Vocal cord nodules and polyps
Food getting stuck in throat	Lung cancer
Lump-in-the-throat sensation	Recurrent leukoplakia
Intermittent airway obstruction	Polypoid degeneration
Chronic airway obstruction	Laryngomalacia
Abdominal bloating	COPD (chronic obstructive
Nasal congestion	Pulmonary disease)
Noisy breathing	Croup
Stridor	Sudden infant death syndrome
Nausea	Sinusitis and allergic symptoms
Snoring	Asthma
	Sleep apnea
	Chronic bronchitis
	Aspiration pneumonia
	Idiopathic pulmonary fibrosis
	Community-acquired pneumonia
	Pneumonia (or recurrent pneumonia)

† Note: In this table the two columns, "Symptoms" and "Conditions," are independent of each other; a symptom on the same line as a condition (and vice versa) does *not* imply correlation.

Although I cannot discuss all of these conditions in this chapter, I will comment on the most important ones: postnasal drip, allergies, sinus disease, asthma, bronchitis, chronic cough, and chronic obstructive pulmonary disease (COPD). I will also briefly discuss the relationship between reflux and aerodigestive tract cancers, cancers of the mouth, larynx (vocal cords), esophagus, and lungs.

> **Nocturnal reflux is the worst kind of reflux pattern because damaging acids and digestive enzymes can remain in contact with the tissues for many hours.**

The nighttime refluxer may only have daytime symptoms, and those are the symptoms that get all the attention. Therefore, one of the great problems with respiratory reflux is that it may go undetected.

Because reflux causes tissue inflammation, changes may be seen on the lining membranes of any or all the parts of the respiratory system and esophagus. The inflamed lining membranes typically increase mucus production. If nighttime reflux enters the nose, nasal congestion and postnasal drip during the day can easily develop and be mistaken for allergies. Believe it or not, nasal congestion is a quite common reflux symptom.

If the lining membranes around the sinus openings swell, sinus symptoms or even actual sinusitis may result. Nevertheless, the underlying cause is reflux. So, reflux-caused symptoms are commonly misdiagnosed as allergies and sinusitis. Among my most frustrated patients are those who previously had ineffective or unnecessary nose and sinus surgery—often multiple surgeries. When their reflux is corrected, their "sinus" symptoms subside.

More about mucus. Under normal conditions, we produce approximately one quart of mucus a day, mostly in the nose. Inflammatory disease of the nose and throat is absolutely characteristic of respiratory reflux; indeed, inflammation results in increased mucus production. It is as if the sick tissue tries to protect itself by manufacturing more mucus, because mucus provides a partial tissue barrier against reflux.

When examining patients, I can often diagnose nocturnal reflux because on examination the patient will demonstrate upper and lower throat findings—so-called *cobblestoning* and *tiger-striping*—that suggest that the refluxate was pooling in certain places in the nose and throat during the night. Those findings are usually associated with an increase in mucus. In fact, thick white mucus on the vocal cords is considered a finding of reflux laryngitis. Such findings, although not well recognized by most physicians, help me accurately diagnose the nighttime refluxer.

Allergies look different than reflux. When examining the nose of the allergic patient, the nasal membranes are swollen and purple and the discharge is thin, watery, and clear. Further, refluxers usually have other throat symptoms whereas patients with allergies do not. It is fairly easy to differentiate reflux from allergies in patients with nasal congestion and postnasal drip.

> **Postnasal drip, chronic throat clearing, excess mucus, sticky throat, lump-in-the-throat sensation, and hoarseness are the most common symptoms of respiratory reflux.**

Breathing problems represent the other significant group of reflux misdiagnoses, the most common being asthma and bronchitis. "Asthma" affects eight percent of Americans (one out of 12) and 17 percent of poor, nonwhite children. We spend in excess of $56 billion a year to treat it. In my book *The Chronic Cough Enigma*,[32] I report that as many as 80 percent of people with asthma are misdiagnosed. Indeed, if that number of "asthma" patients actually has respiratory reflux, then we might save $45 billion a year through accurate diagnosis.

> **The first question to ask anyone with "asthma"—and amazingly, most physicians don't know this—is: When you have trouble breathing during an attack, do you have more difficulty getting air IN or OUT? Trouble during inhalation is due to respiratory reflux, never asthma. Trouble during exhalation is asthma.[29,32]**

How does this work? The difference between breathing IN and OUT is explained by the anatomy and physiology of the airway. With reflux, airway obstruction occurs at the level of the larynx. The upper part of the larynx contains acid receptors, which act like electrical switches. When triggered by exposure to acid, these receptors close the vocal chords, resulting in trouble breathing IN.[12,13,15,29,32] This type of airway obstruction is similar to that seen in children with croup, who may make loud, crowing sounds when breathing IN.

The mechanism of airway obstruction in asthma is completely different. People with asthma have trouble getting air OUT, because breathing tubes within the lungs inside the chest cavity become narrowed. Then, during exhalation, the full lungs exert additional pressure on the already partially collapsed bronchial tubes, resulting in further compression and narrowing. Trying to exhale through such narrowed bronchial tubes leads to prolonged expiration. Noisy breathing during expiration in true asthma is usually called wheezing.

A problem breathing IN is never asthma. Indeed, people with wrong-fully diagnosed asthma don't respond particularly well to asthma treatment, but they do get well when their reflux is controlled. Asthma sufferers and their doctors should know about this.

The next most common respiratory misdiagnoses are chronic cough, bronchitis, and chronic obstructive pulmonary disease (COPD), particularly in nonsmokers.[32] Such patients are usually nocturnal refluxers. Most, but not all, productive ("wet") coughs are due to reflux; although some are actually due to infections or other pulmonary (lung) diseases.

I ask all of my patients to cough out loud to determine if the cough is wet or dry. One can appreciate this by the sound, and most patients know the difference if asked. Generally speaking, a wet cough implies that the reflux goes into the trachea or possibly the lungs at night. For such patients, the cough is usually most productive after the patient arises in the morning.

> **Anyone with chronic bronchitis or even intermittent bronchitis who is a nonsmoker should be evaluated for respiratory reflux.**

People who have pneumonia may very well have reflux aspiration events at night. There appears to be a strong correlation between the findings of nocturnal reflux with massive swelling of the back of the larynx (especially tiger-striping) and wet cough in my respiratory reflux patients. A wet cough by itself is not diagnostic, but the first thing I look for with successful reflux treatment in my patients with respiratory reflux is that the cough is no longer wet.

The final conditions that I wish to discuss here are cancers of the mouth, throat, esophagus, and lungs, all of which may be caused by reflux. My practice is replete with lifelong nonsmokers with tongue, throat, and lung cancer whose reflux was never diagnosed or treated. An item as simple as the Reflux Symptom Index (page 3) might be able to identify respiratory refluxers who are at risk of developing cancer, or if they have had cancer, help to reduce treatment complications and the risk of recurrences.

Twenty-five years ago, I stood at a national meeting and said, "It is my belief that you can get cancer—and I mean all of the aerodigestive cancers, larynx, lung, and esophagus—without smoking, but not without reflux." In the intervening years, I have not changed my mind. Indeed, my clinical experience has confirmed that opinion.

If you have allergies and treatment hasn't helped, think respiratory reflux. If you have sinus disease and surgery hasn't helped, think respiratory reflux. If you have asthma or lung disease (of any type) and the cause is unexplained and/or the treatment ineffective, think respiratory reflux. If you are a nonsmoker or long-time ex-smoker with mouth, throat, or lung cancer, think respiratory reflux. Finally, if you have esophageal cancer (or precancer—i.e., Barrett's esophagus), think (inadequately treated) reflux.

The Cure: Reflux Is Reversible

Reflux need not become chronic, and fortunately for most people, it is correctable. It is useful to understand the pattern and progression of disease that must be altered to allow a person's antireflux defenses to repair the damage and normalize aerodigestive physiology.

Reflux disease is a vicious downward spiral, descending until it seems chronic. Reflux causes reflux, which causes more reflux. Here's the typical scenario: reflux starts for whatever reason—overeating, drinking too much, a late-night binge, the flu—and up come acid and digestive enzymes that inflame healthy tissues.

Unfortunately, the stomach valve itself, the lower esophageal sphincter (LES), which is the most important physiologic barrier preventing stomach contents from escaping into the esophagus, gets swollen and inflamed. With continuing reflux, over time LES function becomes increasingly compromised. Thus, the barrier that is supposed to prevent reflux is damaged, which leads to worsening reflux.

The more one refluxes, the worse esophageal function becomes, until the esophagus is just like a wide-open pipe. Finally, the upper esophageal sphincter (UES), the valve in the lower throat, gives out, so that when the refluxer lies down, everything in the stomach washes into the tunnel-like esophagus and then all the way up into the throat and respiratory tract.

At this stage, esophageal and respiratory reflux occur all night, every night. People with this severity of disease will sometimes wake at night coughing and gasping for air like a fish out of water. This is serious reflux and puts the lungs at risk for aspiration.

But many people with nocturnal reflux sleep right through it, and this explains "silent reflux." People who reflux at night wake in the morning with respiratory symptoms, not digestive symptoms. Indeed, silent reflux has come to mean acid reflux that occurs without heartburn or indigestion.

> To defeat reflux, it takes an all-out effort, with diet and lifestyle changes as the essential therapeutic elements. Just as there is a vicious reflux-causes-reflux cycle progressing downward, cleaning up the problem usually results in an upward spiral toward normalcy.

Yes, normal function of the esophagus and UES can be restored, and diseased respiratory and esophageal tissue can be healed. For more about the cycle of reflux disease, see Chapter 5, "Stages of Reflux and Recovery" (page 29).

Reflux-related respiratory disease, such as misdiagnosed allergies, sinus disease, and asthma can be cured with effective reflux treatment. Even Barrett's esophagus[30-33] can be cured with effective dietary and lifestyle antireflux treatment.[32] For more about that, see *Beyond Barrett's* in "The Longevity Diet" chapter (page 82).

Misconceptions About Reflux

The Internet is a double-edged sword. It is a great source of both information and misinformation. When it comes to reflux, the Internet is remarkably full of nonsense. In this section, I will address five particularly egregious fallacies.

If I take reflux medicine, I can eat whatever I want. Most people, including doctors, mistakenly assume that the primary treatment for reflux disease is acid-suppressive medication. Television advertisements strongly suggest that treatment of heartburn is the goal of antireflux treatment, and that if you take a purple pill, you can eat whatever you want. Unfortunately, nothing could be further from the truth. The goal of antireflux treatment should be to stop reflux and the progression of reflux-caused disease.

The strongest acid-suppressive medications are the proton pump inhibitors (PPIs). These are aggressively marketed, but they should be taken under a doctor's supervision. The belief that PPIs control reflux was turned on its head by a national Danish study of 10,000 patients that concluded that long-term use of PPIs was associated with an increased risk of esophageal cancer.[34] A recent study also found an association between PPIs (though not H2-antagonists) and heart attacks.[35]

When the Danish report came out I was not surprised because the vast majority of my reflux patients come to me already on PPIs, and I knew that PPIs do not control reflux. The esophagus is a very quiet organ, and other than heartburn, it does not complain much. So, symptom relief is not the goal of therapy. The progression of reflux disease in patients taking PPIs goes on unabated. Alleviating just some symptoms is like sweeping dirt under the rug; eventually it will catch up with you.

While the use of acid-suppressive medications is warranted in some patients with reflux, successful treatment and eradication of disease depends more on lifestyle and dietary modifications than on pills.[8] There is even a role for antireflux surgery in highly selected patients, but even laparoscopic fundoplication or other surgeries are doomed to failure without some dietary restraint. The topics of antireflux medication and antireflux surgery are covered in greater detail on pages 41 and 45, respectively.

> This book is a call to action to the medical community to recognize that the most prevalent diseases in America are related to unhealthy diet and lifestyle and that they cannot be cured by pills and procedures.

Some people don't have enough stomach acid. There is a common misperception that some people don't produce enough stomach acid. This is not true. Since 1983, I have been performing reflux testing using a specialized ambulatory acid-sensing device that permits 24-hour pH monitoring. In that time, I have pH tested approximately 15,000 patients, and while there may have been a few people without stomach acid, I cannot recall the last time I came across one.

The exceptions are people who have had certain types of stomach surgery and those with a disease called pernicious anemia. Pernicious anemia is an autoimmune disease in which the lining of the stomach is affected, leaving the person with achlorhydria (no stomach acid). The idea that acid suppression with PPIs might cause pernicious anemia is also false. Pernicious anemia is associated with vitamin B12 deficiency, but antireflux treatment doesn't cause it.

There is another belief that if you take acid-suppressive medications you won't have enough acid to digest your food or to absorb calcium. This is also untrue. PPIs work by inhibiting the cells in the stomach that are responsible for manufacturing stomach acid; but figuratively, if you took handfuls of PPIs every day, you would produce half a ton instead of a ton of acid a day. No acid-suppressive medicine suppresses all of your acid.

Some people have nonacid (bile) reflux. There is no credible evidence that people have nonacid reflux, with the exception of patients who have had their stomachs removed. The suggestion by GI doctors that reflux above pH 4.0 was "nonacid" reflux is not true. Any reflux, even that above pH 4, can damage the respiratory system. The cell biology that was performed in my laboratory over a decade ago showed that acid at pH 5 was damaging to the larynx and vocal cords.[16,22,23,26,27]

I am developing a spit-in-a-cup test for the detection of pepsin (the main stomach enzyme) in the saliva.[23-25] Since pepsin only comes from the stomach, if someone has pepsin in their saliva, they have respiratory reflux. Pepsin in the mouth is pepsin in the airway.

Some acidic foods become alkaline in the body, and some alkaline foods become acidic in the body. This is false. Acid is acid, and alkaline is alkaline. When someone consumes excessive amounts of acid, for example, the excess acid is secreted in the urine, making it more acidic.

Testing one's urine or saliva for acidity is not worthwhile because it has no clinical relevance. It is also important to emphasize that most lists of pH values of foods and beverages on the Internet are confusing and inaccurate. I recommend using pH paper to test common foods that are regularly consumed. For some additional pH food lists, see *Dropping Acid: The Reflux Diet Cookbook & Cure*[1] and www.refluxcookbookblog.com.

Apple cider vinegar (or lemon juice) is good for reflux. One commonly recommended home remedy for heartburn is apple cider vinegar or lemon juice. Perhaps this is based upon the idea that some people don't have enough acid, but for those with respiratory reflux or esophageal reflux, consuming apple cider vinegar or lemon juice is a bad idea.

The entire thrust of this book is that an alkaline diet is important to protect against reflux disease. The scientific evidence and rationale for an alkaline diet is discussed in the next section. In any case, there is not a shred of evidence in the scientific or medical literature that apple cider vinegar is of therapeutic benefit in treating reflux. However, there are reports suggesting that it makes reflux worse.

The best first step you can take to feel better and improve your reflux and your long-term health is to stop consuming acids in any form.

What You Eat Is Eating You: Acid, Pepsin, and All That Jazz

The term *acid reflux* is actually a misnomer because it is the main stomach enzyme, pepsin, which causes tissue inflammation and damage.[1,8,16,22–28,36] Pepsin is also the likely cause of aerodigestive tract cancers.[1,9,22,37,38]

The confusion comes from the fact that pepsin requires acid for its activation. So, instead of calling it *peptic reflux*, I think it is important to explain the cell biology of reflux, or how reflux causes tissue inflammation and how damage occurs.

Until *Dropping Acid: The Reflux Diet Cookbook & Cure*, no one had investigated the adverse effects of the acid in the foods and beverages we consume. Everyone worries about equalizing the stomach's natural acid, yet we continue to pour down ever more acidified foods and drinks. Pepsin can only cause problems when acid is around to activate it.[1,9,16,22] Then it gets busy breaking down proteins into smaller, more easily digestible particles.

Any foods that are high in acid activate pepsin and, if there is no protein around that needs digesting, the pepsin will gnaw on whatever is handy—such as the linings of your throat and esophagus. The old adage "You are what you eat" might in this case be rephrased, "Be careful what you eat, because what you eat could be eating you." Once a pepsin molecule is bound to your throat, for example, *any* dietary source of acid can reactivate it, such as soft drinks, fruit juice, vinegar, or strawberries.

One of the most potent missteps of the FDA resulted in acidification of almost everything packaged in a bottle or can. When they made the *pH less than 4.6 rule*,[1] they never anticipated the consequences.

> Stomach acid is pH 2–4, and today almost every beverage in a bottle or can (except still water) is as acidic as stomach acid; because of this, reflux disease has soared.

I am frequently asked why so many young people have reflux. In 2010, the American Beverage Association reported that the average 12-to-29-year-old American had consumed between 100 and 160 gallons of soda. That amounts to almost a half a gallon per person per day and helps explain why we are currently seeing reflux in 37 percent of young people.[8] For this group, it can be relatively easy to correct the reflux problem—drink water, do not eat late, and avoid junk food and alcohol.

DR. KOUFMAN'S ACID REFLUX DIET

CHAPTER 4
Join the Healthy Revolution

Food and food additives have become a controversial topic in the news. Actually, what's happening is like an insurrection, a rebellion, or a mutiny—a lot of people are unhappy with what's in food these days. America is hopefully on the cusp of major changes in our food supply, and consumers interested in healthy eating appear to be leading the charge. One case in my medical practice exemplifies the contemporary food conflict:

A young woman came to see me with shortness of breath and "asthma." She had trouble getting up a single flight of stairs without huffing and puffing, and she had other symptoms, including postnasal drip, hoarseness, difficulty swallowing, and chronic cough. In addition, her previous sinus surgery had not helped.

Six months after we started working together, she was completely well. Her shortness of breath and "asthma" were gone, and she was off all reflux medicine. She became a healthy eater who had beaten reflux and had lost 32 pounds in the process. As I was telling her that her skin looked great, her eyes looked bright, she looked really healthy, and I knew that she could continue her healthy eating, her husband, who had accompanied her, chimed in, "Well, I don't do any of that; I don't eat healthy . . . and I don't want to."

My patient then gleefully reported that recently her husband had come home with a bucket of fried chicken and all the fixings and announced, "Honey, I brought home dinner." Looking at the bucket and laughing, she responded, "No you didn't!"

This schism is happening across the nation and is part of the problem that many new healthy eaters face with their friends and relatives who aren't. Many patients have trouble modifying their diets and lifestyles if their partners are not supportive.

Meanwhile, the entire question of what actually constitutes healthy eating is becoming a national debate. We have new insight into obesity, diabetes, and reflux disease, and people who care about these issues are beginning to effectively wield both political and economic pressure in important ways.

In 2015, the major restaurant chain, Chipotle, announced that it would no longer serve genetically modified foods; General Mills announced that it would discontinue the use of artificial flavors and colors in breakfast cereals; and the FDA banned the use of trans fats by 2018.

These changes have occurred as the result of consumer pressure, not government action, as the cost of making these changes is estimated at $100 billion for the food industry.

"Generally Recognized as Safe" (GRAS)[1,6-8] is an FDA designation established by the Food Additives Amendment of 1958 that designates a chemical or substance added to food as safe in its intended use and therefore exempted from the usual Federal Food, Drug, and Cosmetic Act (FFDCA) food additive tolerance requirements.

Using this process, the food industry has been able to introduce a variety of chemicals and preservatives—all approved by the FDA—into the food supply. The FDA does not have scientists who check on the safety of ingredients already approved as GRAS. Once an item gets on the approved GRAS list, it rarely comes off.

We now know that the GRAS list of food additives introduced in the 1970s primarily to prolong shelf life never had rigorous scientific scrutiny, and, until now, there was little consideration of unhealthy, long-term consequences.

In 1973, following an outbreak of food poisoning, the FDA regulated foods and beverages in bottles and cans, demanding acidification as a preservative to kill bacteria and prolong shelf life.[1] All such products crossing state lines had to have a pH level of 4.6 or less.[1,8] I am sure that they never dreamed that the food and beverage industry would increase the acidity to remarkably unhealthy levels (pH 2–3).

There is no question that the arc of the reflux and esophageal cancer epidemics mirrors that of soft drink consumption since the 1960s. Too much dietary acid is clearly bad for reflux, and it now appears that it is also bad for bone density.

Yet when I wrote to the FDA asking that they consider including the pH of all canned and bottled beverages on the nutritional label, their response was that "the weight of scientific evidence does not lead us to conclude that acids are harmful." So, what should we wait for? The time when esophageal cancer affects half of the population? When will there be enough disease data to put pH labeling on foods?

> Find a way to voice your support: write to your representatives in Congress and to the Food and Drug Administration and ask them to put the pH (acidity) of all canned and bottled foods and beverages on the nutritional label.

Food (Sugar) Addiction

How did we get so unhealthy in the first place? One answer is our consumption of trans fat, sugar, and bread, all of which are addictive. *Bread,* you ask? As you will see in the section *Pick Your Poison or Cure* (page 75), flour changed in the 1960s, and bread became sugar—and excess sugar becomes fat.[2–5]

Many Americans are addicted to sugar, and we became addicted to sugary soft drinks, snack foods, and bread at about the same time. Diet soft drinks were not popular in the 1970s and 1980s when the obesity epidemic started to explode. And we love bread. We eat bread for breakfast, lunch, dinner, and snacks. Sugar is everywhere; it is in almost everything we consume. America's addiction to sugar is the main cause of obesity and diabetes today.[2]

I went to the largest grocery store I could find, and the cereal aisle stretched as far as the eye could see. After 30 minutes of searching, I was unable to find a single breakfast cereal that did not contain sugar. I bet there were 10,000 boxes of cereal on those shelves. I asked the store manager if they carried any cereals that didn't contain sugar. The answer was no, although there were a handful that had "reduced sugar."

How ubiquitous is sugar in our diets? Go to your supermarket and look at the ingredients of the most common foods you purchase, including condiments, soups, broths, canned goods, and baked goods. You may be surprised to find that almost all of them contain sugar and, in many cases, sugar is listed as a main ingredient, at or near the top of the ingredient list.

> There is sugar in 80 percent of the products in your grocery store, and in most products, it is extra sugar added for sweetening.

While breaking sugar addiction is not the first concern for *Dr. Koufman's Acid Reflux Diet*, it is a crucial variable in the fight against disease. If you are obese, you need to consider removing all refined sugar from your diet and getting sugar, albeit reduced amounts, from complex carbohydrates and fruit instead. In the section *Pick Your Poison or Cure* (page 75), I outline some strategies for breaking sugar addiction.

It appears that overcoming food addiction is very much like quitting smoking or quitting drinking alcohol. In fact, the Alcoholics Anonymous model seems to apply especially well to sugar addiction. It is possible to break it, but for many the process is painful and, as with smoking and alcoholism, there is a risk of relapsing.

Whether you are young or old, you should begin to think about health maintenance, disease prevention, and healthy eating. Let this book be your opportunity to begin the process, which will demand close scrutiny of your diet and lifestyle. And, if you have a partner, they need to be involved if you are to succeed. *Dr. Koufman's Acid Reflux Diet* is designed to make a big difference.

Eat Lean, Clean, Green, and Alkaline

The major dietary and lifestyle changes of *Dr. Koufman's Acid Reflux Diet* are summarized here. You can copy this page and put it on your refrigerator, carry it in your pocket, or send it to friends.

1. Eat 75 percent of your calories before 5:00 p.m. and your last meal of the day at least four hours before bedtime. Try to close the kitchen by 8:00 p.m., but 7:00 p.m. is even better.

2. Avoid bad trans fats by reading food labels, and limit your consumption of butter and red meat.

3. Avoid all processed and fast foods. If the package label on the food or beverage contains ingredients that are unknown or that you cannot pronounce, consider them poison and eliminate those items from your diet permanently.

4. Stop drinking all soft drinks—including store-bought fruit juices, sports drinks, energy drinks, vitamin waters, and seltzer. They are all too acidic. Your healthy choices? Drink water—alkaline water with a pH higher than 8.5 is best[31]—and drink coffee and tea in moderation, though not bottled brands, as they contain added acid too.

5. Limit your intake of highly acidic fruits and foods, including citrus fruit, canned sauces, and bottled or canned fruit.

6. Always add your own condiments, salad dressings, sauces, and cheeses—that is, when eating out, ask for condiments *on the side* so you can add them yourself in moderation.

7. Plan ahead and bring food to work. You will need healthy food in your refrigerator at work as well as at home.

8. Know your limits—don't overeat—and know the trigger foods that cause you to have reflux.

9. Alcohol is a major reflux trigger for many people. At the very least, no late-night drinking and especially no nightcaps. Big drinkers usually have big reflux. If alcohol is a trigger for your reflux, you may need to quit drinking altogether.

10. The best foods are fish, poultry, salads, fruits and vegetables, healthy nuts, grains, tubers, rice, and eggs. Special mention goes to bananas, melons, ginger, fennel, avocados, parsley, and greens.

At the beginning of this section, I implied that *Dr. Koufman's Acid Reflux Diet* is intuitive and sensible. But intuition depends on analysis and good information. Take some time for careful self-analysis and consider the following questions:

Am I overweight? Am I obese?

Am I a food addict, and if so, to which foods? Sugar?

Do I eat a healthy breakfast and lunch each and every day?

Do I have unhealthy dietary habits, such as eating too late?

Do I eat too much junk food and/or drink too many soft drinks?

Do I drink (alcohol) too much or drink too late?

Do I eat dinner too late?

Each of these questions will need to be addressed if you are going to be successful.

CHAPTER 5

Stages of Reflux and Recovery

de·com·pen·sa·tion *n.* the functional deterioration of a previously
working structure or system.

P eople often ask me, what is the best treatment for reflux? The answer
is there is no one best treatment because reflux comes in many forms
and affects people very differently at different times. Treatment
must be individualized.

For a physician specializing in treating reflux patients, the reflux-treatment algorithm is huge. I have a complex mosaic of treatment options
from which a customized program is fashioned for each and every patient.
The key is accurate pre-treatment assessment and diagnosis.

If you have been taking a PPI medication for years, the idea that there
is no one-size-fits-all treatment may be a surprise to you, but different
treatment elements are necessary at different stages of every patient's reflux
disease.

The suggestion that there are different stages of reflux is in line with
our understanding of other diseases. Even common upper respiratory infections like a cold or the flu have stages: a prodrome (sneezing, nasal congestion, and runny nose), followed by the acute phase (fever, malaise, sore
throat, cough, etc.), followed by the recovery phase, which is sometimes
followed by complications such as sinusitis or bronchitis. Reflux has different stages as well.

How serious is your reflux? People with indigestion once or twice a
month after overeating rarely seek medical attention, but those with daily,
life-disrupting symptoms do. And the symptoms that bring people to see
me are frightening respiratory symptoms—trouble breathing is not a symptom that can be ignored, nor is chest pain that mimics a heart attack, or a

violent cough that disrupts normal daily life. As you will see, symptom frequency and severity are not the only variables in this equation; the stage of an individual's reflux also depends on co-morbidities such as obesity and other conditions that alter the resilience of the body's antireflux defenses.

In *The Cure: Reflux Is Reversible* (pages 15–17), I suggest that severe reflux usually follows a cascade of events, a downward spiral: as reflux worsens, it further impairs antireflux defenses so that reflux begets more reflux. Although this book was written primarily for refluxers who are *not* in the acute phase but who have already battled reflux and now seek long-term dietary solutions, in this chapter I will explain the mechanisms and processes of decompensation and of recovery.

The fact that reflux is not a static condition and thus sufferers differ widely is both a problem and an opportunity. The problem is that people experience such different patterns of reflux, with different reflux trigger foods and different responses to different therapies at different times. But the opportunity lies in the ability to assess where you stand and then make all of the correct adjustments. The chapters that follow discuss the four phases of *Dr. Koufman's Acid Reflux Diet*: detox, transition, maintenance, and longevity. Where do you fit, and where do you start? The answer will depend upon the stage of your reflux and variables that are unique to you.

The Four Stages of Reflux

IV. Acute (decompensated)

III. Brittle (partly compensated)

II. Stable (but still vulnerable)

I. Remission (compensated)

In my experience, there are four stages or phases of reflux, but they form a continuum. People need different levels of treatment depending on their stage, but generally people with Stages III or IV need medical attention.

Stage IV, or decompensation, implies that the patient is unable to recover on her or his own and that intervention must be customized and focused on all of the parts of the reflux system that are dysfunctional. For Stage IV patients, I usually perform reflux testing including esophageal function testing.[1,9,18,32]

Stage III, or brittle, patients are out of the abyss of decompensation, but still on the edge. The word *brittle* implies that it would not take much for them to regress, so they must pay close attention to all of the therapeutic elements, especially the diet. Brittle refluxers are at the beginning of the transition phase (page 53), and as they add foods back into their diets following the reflux detox period, they still must avoid high-risk foods such as chocolate, fatty meats, and alcohol. Stage III extends from the end of detox until Stage II. For some people, overcoming Stage III takes weeks, and for others it can take months.

Stage II, or stable but still vulnerable, implies that the patient's symptoms are under control and that they are near remission. *Remission* implies that trigger foods have been identified and are avoided and that medical treatment may be successfully tapered if the patient is still taking any reflux medications. Stage II patients are usually feeling confident about their reflux and health although they still have to plan meals and dining out.

Stage I, or remission, is the goal. This is the stage when people go about their lives without excessive day-to-day concerns for dietary and lifestyle issues. It does not imply, however, that relapse could never occur. When people are in remission, they still must pay close attention to how they eat when out of their regular routine, such as when traveling to a foreign country.

You will need to figure out where you are on this continuum before you embark on your reflux-rehabilitation program. Otherwise, you will not know where to start. In my opinion, when in doubt, start with the strict, two-week reflux detox program (page 47).

Before expanding the stages of reflux in the context of its physiology and pathology, I would like to explain the process of decompensation. I wrote my laws of decompensation long ago in reference to voice disorders, but they apply equally well to reflux.

The Laws of Decompensation

1st Axiom: Before—the components of a system are in dynamic balance.
1st Corollary: Conflicting elements are held together by function and purpose.

2nd Axiom: Decompensation is preceded by often-ignored warning signs.
2nd Corollary: During early destabilization, imbalance is assessable.

3rd Axiom: Last-straw principle: When threshold is exceeded, collapse occurs.
3rd Corollary: Recovery requires repair and stabilization of all elements.

The laws of decompensation apply to many things in life that appear to happen slowly, even silently, then all of a sudden. (Such events even include dissimilar things like divorce and the failure of a business.)

I include the laws of decompensation here because they reveal my clinical approach to diagnosis and treatment. In my practice, virtually all decompensated patients undergo reflux testing, as well as patients who are not responding to treatment in a timely fashion.

The laws of decompensation form an arc, just like reflux and its treatment, with repair of all essential elements required before dynamic balance can be restored—before the reflux system is again working properly. Let's work from health to disease by first examining Stage I, normal physiology.

Before—the components of a system are in dynamic balance

After you take a bite of food and begin to chew, you form a ball of food called a bolus (from the Latin for "ball") with your tongue. Once you initiate a swallow, an automatic sequence begins. These synchronized events allow you to pass the bolus from the mouth into the throat, then into the esophagus, and down to and into the stomach.

The autonomic nervous system, run by the vagus nerve, is the driver of this entire sequence. As a model, consider the reflux system as if it were a machine: it is a one-piston, two-valve system with a conveyor belt between the two valves, one at the top and one at the bottom.

The tongue thrust and the pharyngeal (throat) part of the swallow compose the piston. The upper esophageal sphincter (UES) and the lower esophageal sphincter (LES) are the two valves, and the conveyor belt is the esophagus, that muscular tube that connects the throat at the UES to the stomach at the LES.

Once the bolus enters the throat, the swallow is initiated when the tongue muscles push downward and the muscular walls of the pharynx contract, driving the bolus to the upper edge of the UES. Incidentally, during this part of the swallow, the larynx (voice box) automatically clamps shut so that nothing swallowed gets into the trachea or lungs below.

When the bolus reaches the UES, the UES should promptly open, allowing the bolus to pass. After it passes, the UES should close behind it. At that point, peristalsis, a series of muscular contractions of the esophagus, begins pushing the bolus down the esophagus toward the LES, which should open in a timely fashion to allow the bolus to enter the stomach. After it passes the LES, the valve should close. As you will see, Stage IV refluxers often have problems with both valves and the conveyer belt.

Conflicting elements are held together by function and purpose

This synchronized swallow that transports the bolus from the mouth to the stomach is only half the story. Keeping the bolus and all the other stomach contents in the stomach and protecting the aerodigestive tract against reflux is another task of the system. There are four primary antireflux defenses.[9]

The first defense is the LES, which is the primary barrier against gastroesophageal reflux, the movement of stomach contents from the stomach into the esophagus. The LES is imperfect, and through pH-monitoring studies we know that a healthy person can have up to 50 reflux episodes a day without having reflux disease—that is, without having esophageal or respiratory reflux symptoms and findings.[9] These "physiologic reflux" episodes are generally short-lived, mostly occurring after meals. Keeping physiologic reflux from progressing to reflux disease is the purpose of the antireflux defenses. In normalcy, the LES must work most of the time; otherwise reflux disease will result.

The second defense, called *esophageal acid clearance,* is the ability of the esophagus to clear the refluxate (that which was refluxed) and reestablish normal, nonacidic pH after any reflux event has occurred. This defense also involves a sequence.

A reflux event is normally followed by several automatic swallows, which help normalize the esophageal pH. The first swallow clears the bolus of the refluxate back into the stomach. Then, additional swallows deliver saliva, which contains acid-neutralizing bicarbonate. Bicarbonate, secreted by normal saliva glands, is the opposite of acid, and the swallowed saliva with bicarbonate neutralizes any remaining acid on the surface lining of the tubular esophagus.

The clearing of normal esophageal acid depends on the presence of saliva. People who have dry mouth from any cause almost always have reflux disease. One example that is easily overlooked is radiation therapy for head and neck cancer. While these tumors are not particularly common, radiation therapy is often part of the overall treatment program. Unfortunately, radiation results in almost complete destruction of the saliva glands and loss of salivary bicarbonate.

A lack of saliva, called *xerostomia,* is associated with reflux in virtually all patients following radiation of the saliva glands. In other words, the neutralization that is supposed to occur following a physiologic reflux event cannot occur without salivary bicarbonate. Therefore, any person who has had radiation, or even anyone who has terrible dry mouth—the other condition that causes xerostomia is Sjogren's syndrome—should take precautions to prevent developing reflux.[9] Indeed, they should be on a permanent alkaline diet, specifically one similar to the diet presented in *Beyond Barrett's* (page 84) in "The Longevity Diet" chapter.

The third antireflux defense is a unique way the esophagus is able to defend itself. Other than the saliva glands, the esophagus is the only other organ that can manufacture and secrete bicarbonate. Bicarbonate, however, does not neutralize pepsin, and this esophageal defense can be overwhelmed and become ineffective if there is too much reflux—that is, more than 50 reflux events per day.[9]

The fourth and most important defense against respiratory reflux is the UES. Anatomically, the UES is made up of a muscular sling from the voice box and pharynx that goes around the uppermost part of the esophagus. Under normal circumstances, the UES prevents reflux from exiting the esophagus and coming up into the pharynx and the respiratory tract. But severe reflux, particularly nocturnal reflux, can render the UES completely ineffective as a barrier.

Decompensation is preceded by often-ignored warning signs

In people with respiratory and/or esophageal reflux, different parts of the usually coordinated antireflux defenses may be impaired. Understanding the sequence of how things go wrong, how the different parts of the system stop working, is useful. As a clinician, my first step is to identify the broken parts because knowing precisely which parts are not working usually explains why a person has certain symptoms and helps me choose the right treatment.

The vast majority of my patients are already decompensated (Stage IV) and typically have many symptoms. Occasionally, some patients have just one symptom, such as postnasal drip (having had unsuccessful treatment for allergies or sinusitis) or hoarseness (having had unsuccessful voice therapy). Stage IV patients will often report having had several different symptoms, often intermittently for many years.

Let me emphasize that all of the symptoms shown in the Reflux Symptom Index quiz (page 3) may be the result of respiratory reflux. Pay attention to your symptoms, even the minor ones, and think about the possibility of respiratory reflux even if you have no digestive symptoms such as heartburn or indigestion.

There is another totally different and objective scoring system for the throat examination, called the Reflux Finding Score (RFS).[1,11,14,17] Points are awarded for each specific finding such as vocal cord swelling, swelling of the back of the larynx (tiger-striping), mucus on the vocal cords, erythema (redness), narrowing of the airway, and so on. The RFS is the sum of 10 different items.[1]

A normal RFS is 0–3. A score of 4–9 is mild-to-moderate reflux. A score of 10 is considered "reflux purgatory"—that is, the number between not severe and severe. A score of 11–15 is considered moderately severe, and a score of over 16 is considered very severe. About half of my patients present with scores of 14–17, and fewer than 10 percent of my patients present with scores of 18 or more. Typically those patients have significant trouble breathing and often many other distressing symptoms as well.

It is equally important to understand that as patients get well and the RFS falls toward the normal range, antireflux medications can be tapered and stopped. Indeed, for patients who may be on PPIs, those medicines are usually discontinued when the RFS is 8 or less.

During early destabilization, imbalance is assessable

The throat, especially the larynx, is a barometer of the entire reflux system. The RFS is a quantitative method for assessing respiratory reflux, and I can determine the relative severity of respiratory reflux and whether the reflux is daytime, nighttime, or both just by examining the throat.

In nocturnal refluxers, the back of the larynx will often be swollen to the point that it touches the back wall of the throat. I call this finding *tiger-striping* because that is what it resembles. Longtime nocturnal refluxers usually also have changes in the back of the nose that I call *cobblestoning*, as well as granularity in the narrowing of the entire pharynx (throat). In addition, I can usually tell which patients snore and have sleep apnea by the throat examination. Indeed, the entire tube of the throat is granular and very narrow in these patients.

Sometimes patients with relatively minor symptoms in fact have severe reflux. They might be minimizing or denying their symptoms, or they might be nighttime refluxers who have not yet decompensated.

It is beyond the scope of this book to discuss all of the laryngeal findings of respiratory reflux. However, you should know that a skilled clinician, particularly an ENT doctor, can make the diagnosis of reflux based upon the symptoms and throat examination.

Last-straw principle: When threshold is exceeded, collapse occurs

There are many factors that can precipitate decompensation. These include an upper respiratory infection, intense emotional stress, weight gain, vacation (especially travel with late-night eating), and a change in diet. I am also amazed at how many patients date the onset of worsening reflux to a trendy diet.

Here are **five red flags** associated with reflux decompensation.

1. New breathing problems or worsening of an existing one. Any change in breathing, including asthma-like symptoms, shortness of breath, choking episodes, gasping for air in the night, chronic cough, or discomfort taking a full breath. Any of these are signs that the respiratory reflux is severe. All "reactive airways diseases" should be considered Stage IV reflux until proven otherwise.

2. Difficulty swallowing or painful swallowing. A very common manifestation of respiratory reflux is discoordination (impairment) of the swallowing mechanism. The UES may go into spasm. For example, I saw a man with severe reflux who had great difficulty swallowing, so I performed special testing (pharyngeal/UES/esophageal manometry), which showed that his resting UES pressure was 240 mmHg (millimeters of mercury pressure). To better understand what this means: If your blood pressure reached this number, you would be admitted to the hospital. Or consider how your arm feels when your blood pressure is checked and your arm is squeezed above 200 mmHg. It hurts. That's how tight this man's UES was, and it was closing during the middle of his swallow.

Painful swallowing is an even more ominous symptom, particularly when there is referred pain that goes up into the ear. This demands a prompt examination, as throat cancer is a possibility.

3. Development of chronic cough (more than eight weeks' duration). Development of a chronic cough—a duration of more than eight weeks—particularly a wet, productive cough, suggests severe respiratory reflux. Coughing up mucus, especially in the morning, is usually a manifestation of nighttime reflux that falls into the trachea, the large breathing tube just below the vocal cords, or even further down into the bronchial tubes and lungs. Chronic cough, tracheitis, and bronchitis result from respiratory reflux, and the development of those conditions in a nonsmoker should be considered respiratory reflux until proven otherwise.

4. Hoarseness or laryngitis. Any voice change in a nonsmoker should be considered reflux-related, unless the person has an ongoing respiratory infection at the time, such as a cold. Physicians often don't connect voice change with reflux, but respiratory reflux is the single most common cause of hoarseness. "Whiskey voice," or morning hoarseness after a night of drinking, is absolutely characteristic of reflux. But even if you don't drink, if you awaken with morning hoarseness, the chances still are that you had reflux during the night.

5. Prolonged upper respiratory infection. Upper respiratory infections (URIs) can trigger reflux decompensation. Think about it this way: the lining membranes of the respiratory tract were marginally able to withstand some ongoing reflux until a respiratory infection further compromised their integrity. Most cold and flu viruses damage the nose and throat lining, which then weakens antireflux defenses. It's easy to imagine how a respiratory infection might lead to worsening reflux. Indeed, if you have persistent symptoms weeks or months after an upper respiratory infection, think respiratory reflux.

What characterizes decompensation and the decompensated patient? Are you a Stage IV reflux patient?

If you have daily symptoms

If your symptoms are disrupting your life

If your symptoms demand medical attention

If you have any breathing symptoms—including "allergies" or "asthma"—and you are not getting better with treatment

. . . then you probably have reflux and you are Stage IV, decompensation. If you have taken the Reflux Symptom Index quiz (page 3) and your score is more than 25, you most certainly are Stage IV.

The cascade of events that causes decompensation is succinctly presented in the section *The Cure: Reflux Is Reversible* (page 15). The worse your reflux, the more you will reflux until it is impossible to correct the problem without an all-out effort.

For most Stage IV refluxers, dietary and lifestyle modifications alone are sometimes not enough. Patients who are in the decompensated state can try the two-week reflux detox diet, but medical intervention targeting the specific elements of the damaged reflux system is often needed as well.

Recovery requires stabilization and repair of all essential elements

Typically, decompensated patients come to me already on a PPI and with a modified diet, having already read *Dropping Acid: The Reflux Diet Cookbook & Cure*, yet they are still suffering. These patients require a comprehensive evaluation of the entire digestive tract that may include reflux testing, swallowing evaluation, transnasal esophagoscopy (TNE),[30,32] and even neuromuscular testing of the vagus nerve.[39]

At the Voice Institute of New York, I perform reflux testing for every patient with Stage IV reflux because specific information is needed to determine the proper treatment regimen. In the typical Stage IV patient, the RFS for the laryngeal examination is 16, and manometry demonstrates poor esophageal peristaltic function as well as poor esophageal valve function. pH monitoring shows extensive daytime and nighttime reflux in both the pharynx and esophagus. All of those findings are important because treatment must restore esophageal and esophageal valve function, and acid-suppression pills alone are often not enough.[1,8,19,34]

> Most decompensated Stage IV patients have nocturnal reflux; therefore, planning an early dinner no later than 6 p.m. going forward will be essential.

My therapeutic programs are always customized, and for many patients treatment will be altered depending on their progress after initiation of treatment. For example, most patients on antireflux medications will have those medications reduced or stopped within weeks to months, when they show improvement on their RFS examinations.

I recognize that after having read this section, you may still be uncertain as to what stage of reflux you are in. In truth, unless you undergo medical examination and reflux testing, you'll have to judge by your symptoms. Be aware that most people with respiratory reflux minimize the severity of their symptoms until decompensation. If you have chronic postnasal drip and morning hoarseness, consider that you are likely a Stage III or IV refluxer, and all people at Stage III or IV need to start with the reflux detox program (page 47).

For those of you with milder symptoms, view the entire reflux diet program as a healthy longevity diet. I recognize that most people will pick and choose among the options and recommendations, but there are some absolutes. The two biggest are *no soft drinks* and *no night eating*.

Why an Alkaline Diet?

The rationale for this diet being alkaline is based on science, particularly research on the enzyme pepsin[1,9,28] and cell biology,[16,22,23,26,27] the impact of reflux at the cellular level, as well as my 35 years of clinical experience. In a nutshell, the goals of this reflux diet are to deactivate and wash out tissue-bound pepsin, and restore normal antireflux defenses and normal aerodigestive tract physiology.

The stages of reflux—acute, or decompensated; brittle, or partly compensated; stable but still vulnerable; and remission, or compensated—form a continuum from very bad to very good. The four stages are not time-locked, and sometimes they overlap and go back and forth. If so, the two-week reflux detox diet can be extended for many weeks, or even months. For most people, however, the detox period is two to four weeks, since control of reflux in the first phase is designed to break the cascade that caused decompensation.

The transition phase of the diet follows the detox program. Foods are reintroduced into the patient's diet, and this phase is characterized by trial and error. The transition phase can last up to a year because it takes that long for some people to discover all the trigger foods that set off their reflux. Remember, everyone is different. For every patient who can eat green peppers but not red peppers, there is another who can eat red but not green. However, despite individual differences, there are certain admonitions that are steadfast throughout all phases of *Dr. Koufman's Acid Reflux Diet*, such as the ban on overly acidic foods and beverages.

The maintenance phase assumes that an individual can manage his or her own reflux as long as disciplined planning and vigilance are applied. As you will see, making meal plans is a good idea during the maintenance phase, ideally planning a week in advance. At last, remission!

Antireflux Medication

I do not want to leave the impression that I don't use medications to treat reflux patients. In fact, since most of my patients present to me in Stage IV, I use a lot of medications to help restore normal function of the reflux system. Nevertheless, diet and lifestyle modifications are the most important elements of treatment. People who think that antireflux medication is the cure are sadly mistaken.

> **Antireflux medication is an adjunctive therapy to dietary and lifestyle modifications, and not the other way around.**

The two main types of acid-suppressive medications that are most prescribed by doctors and used by patients (most are available over-the-counter) are proton pump inhibitors (PPIs) and H2-antagonists (H2As). PPIs are stronger; however, they have a much worse side-effect profile, and in my opinion, they should not be taken without physician supervision. When PPIs are stopped abruptly, reflux may get much worse; this is called rebound hyperacidity. In addition, the side effects of PPIs are common and include diarrhea, abdominal pain, and bloating. Conversely, H2As are safe and effective, they have few side effects, and they can be used on an as-needed basis (not so with PPIs).

Classes and Brands of Commonly Used Antireflux Medications
Brand names in parentheses

Proton pump inhibitors (PPIs)	omeprazole† (Prilosec)
	pantaprazole† (Protonix)
	esomeprazole† (Nexium)
	dexlansoprazole (Dexilant)
	omeprazole/bicarb (Zegerid)
	lansoprazole† (Prevacid)
	rabeprazole† (Acifex)
H2-antagonists (H2As)	famotidine† (Pepcid)
	cimetidine† (Tagamet)
Prokinetic agents	domperidone† (Motilium)
	metoclopramide (Reglan)
	erythromycin†
Neuropathic syndrome meds	gabapentin† (Neurontin)
	pregabalin† (Lyrica)
	amitriptyline† (Elavil)
Miscellaneous	liquid alginate† (Gaviscon Advance Aniseed)

This list is not intended to be complete. I have indicated those medications that I use in my practice with the dagger (†) symbol.

Who needs medication? A typical case was a 32-year-old man who worked on Wall Street. Thin, athletic, and hard-working, he often worked long hours and then went out eating and drinking with co-workers after 10 p.m. Reflux testing revealed that he had severe nighttime reflux into both the esophagus and the respiratory tract. On manometry, his UES was weak, and he had a lazy esophagus—that is, impaired esophageal peristalsis.

I placed this patient on the two-week reflux detox diet shown on page 47—nothing out of a bottle or can except alkaline water, no eating within four hours of bed, and no alcohol. In addition, he was started on a PPI in the morning with H2-antagonists before lunch, dinner, and bed. I did not initially treat the esophageal dysmotility on the assumption that when his reflux improved so too would his esophageal motility and esophageal valve function. They did.

Six weeks later, his reflux was under control, and I started to deescalate his medicines, discontinuing the PPI first. Subsequently, I performed an esophageal examination (TNE), and found he had Barrett's esophagus (see *Beyond Barrett's,* page 82). I then put him on a long-term alkaline diet, and he willingly changed his lifestyle and stopped drinking alcohol completely.

I explain the difference between PPIs and H2As above; here I will discuss the last three classes of medication in the table.

Prokinetic agents are medications that specifically target improving esophageal function, both motility and valve function. They are not used routinely.

Detailed explanations of *neuropathic syndromes*[32,40] and the medications used to treat them are beyond the scope of this book, but a word about neuropathic syndromes is needed. The word *neuropathic* means "nerve-caused" or "sick-nerve syndrome," and neuropathic symptoms are common in reflux patients.

The powerful vagus nerve (the Xth cranial nerve) dominates the aerodigestive tract. The vagus is the motor and sensory nerve for the throat, voice, esophagus, intestines, and liver, and it even sends branches to the heart and ear. The vagus nerve runs from the skull, in the back of the throat (just under the lining membrane) and then down into the chest. If the vagus nerve is damaged in any way—the most common causes are a nasty throat virus that infects the nerve, and trauma, some kind of physical injury to the nerve itself—then neuropathic symptoms may result.[32,40]

The most common neuropathic symptoms are painful speaking, burning throat, and chronic cough. Using specialized testing (laryngeal electromyography[39]), vagal neuropathic syndromes can be definitively diagnosed. These symptoms and syndromes can be treated with medications that affect the vagus nerve, but I use these medications only when needed to ameliorate neuropathic symptoms. My book *The Chronic Cough Enigma* discusses neuropathic syndromes in greater detail.[32]

> Painful speaking, burning throat, and chronic cough are typically neurogenic symptoms that may or may not resolve with reflux control alone.

The last medication, *liquid alginate*, is very popular for reflux treatment in Europe but not in the U.S. The reason is that the brand that I recommend (liquid Gaviscon Advance Aniseed) is not found in our drug stores but is available on-line.

Alginates, derived from seaweed, are not really medication in the sense that people do not seem to have drug reactions to them. Alginates are unique in the reflux-treatment armamentarium; they form a "raft" within the stomach at the bottom of the LES that helps block reflux, particularly nighttime reflux. I recommend that my patients with nocturnal reflux take Gaviscon (the U.K. product, not the U.S. version) before bed.

Since their introduction in the 1980s, PPIs have become big business for Big Pharma. Currently, we spend billions every year on PPIs. Unfortunately, these medications are not a panacea, and we now know that they do not control the progression of reflux disease.[8,19,34]

For the last decade, I have been backing away from their long-term use, but I do use them at the beginning of treatment in most decompensated patients. It is usually the first medication discontinued, and often it can be discontinued within the first six to eight weeks.

> If you have been taking PPIs for years, you probably should get off them; consult your doctor and consider better treatment alternatives.

A word of caution about discontinuing PPIs: stopping them abruptly with no medication replacement can result in rebound hyperacidity and acute worsening of reflux symptoms. For tapering, I replace PPIs with H2-antagonists four times a day (before each meal and at bedtime). After a week or so, the H2As can usually be deescalated as well, one mealtime pill less every few days. Sometimes, I add Gaviscon Advance after each meal and before bed for patients with significant rebound symptoms; usually the H2As and the Gaviscon can be tapered within a few weeks.

Antireflux Surgery

There are antireflux surgical procedures designed to improve function of the LES. Most of the newer "minimally invasive" procedures are ineffective and/or dangerous. The one procedure that I do recommend is called the Stretta procedure.[41–43] Unfortunately, some health insurance companies do not yet cover its cost, even though when compared to traditional antireflux surgery, it saves an average of $10,000 per procedure.

Stretta is actually not a true surgical procedure, as there is no "cutting," and it is performed in an endoscopy suite with mild sedation. To perform Stretta, a special instrument is inserted into the esophagus, and the LES is treated with non-ablative, low-power, and low-temperature radiofrequency energy.[42] Months later the LES appears thickened and stronger. The advantages of Stretta are that it has been effective in 80 percent of my patients, and it does not prohibit the future use of any other treatment options. I recommend Stretta for patients who have demonstrated poor LES function and who have continuing reflux despite aggressive treatment including a healthy diet and lifestyle.

Real surgery? The antireflux surgical procedure that has stood the test of time is called laparoscopic fundoplication.[44] It is performed in a hospital operating room by a surgeon. Small holes are made in the abdomen to insert laparoscopic instruments, and the dome of the stomach is loosened, wrapped around the esophagus, and sutured to create a tight angle so that food going into the stomach does not come back out.

This surgery is a last resort, but I do recommend it for patients with respiratory reflux whose lungs are compromised. For that subgroup of respiratory refluxers, laparoscopic fundoplication can be lifesaving.[32]

When and Why Should I See a Doctor?

Anyone who has had reflux symptoms for years, even intermittently, should be seen by a physician. This recommendation may surprise you since this book is about how to treat reflux with a healthy diet and lifestyle. However, the reality is that the development of esophageal cancer may be relatively silent, and it is now more common than ever. Indeed, in terms of its incidence, according to the National Cancer Institute, it is the fastest growing cancer in America.[32,45]

People who have reflux should undergo throat and esophageal examinations if they have had reflux for several years, and especially if they have been taking PPIs. You no longer need to be anesthetized in a special facility to have an endoscopy.

Transnasal esophagoscopy[30] (TNE) is the superior alternative. It is performed with the patient awake and sitting upright while an ultrathin endoscope is passed through the nose. TNE gives a superior examination, and unlike sedated endoscopy, TNE does not require any recovery time. Since there is no anesthesia other than numbing of the nose, the patient does not need to be accompanied by another person, and can return to normal activities immediately after the procedure.

TNE is comfortable, is well tolerated, and is done during a regular doctor visit. In my opinion, TNE is the best first examination of the esophagus for all refluxers. So, if you have had reflux symptoms for years, you should have your esophagus checked. TNE is safer, less expensive, and more accurate than sedated GI endoscopy. For more information, see www.transnasalesophagoscopy.com.

CHAPTER 6

Two-Week Reflux Detox

With over a decade's experience using a two-week reflux detox diet, I can attest that over half of the patients notice a big difference after those two weeks. The most important elements are the timing and size of meals.

Although I recommend no eating, drinking, or lying down within four hours of bed, I also recommend that the evening meal be consumed before 7 p.m. As the day goes on, the reflux system appears to slow. So, a meal finished at 8 p.m., with bedtime around midnight, may still be associated with nocturnal reflux. I emphasize this point because nocturnal reflux tends to be far more damaging than daytime reflux, even if you sleep soundly through the night. Remember, during sleep, acid and pepsin can remain in contact with your respiratory tract and esophageal tissues for many hours.

The "dropping acid" element of the diet is crucial, and so is drinking alkaline water. Pepsin requires acid for activation, and alkaline water with a pH of 8.0 or higher actually neutralizes pepsin; it destroys the pepsin molecule.[31] The diet does not permit consumption of anything in a bottle or can except water, because almost everything else that is bottled is acidic. In addition, the only fruits allowed during detox are melons and bananas. Finally, no known reflux-causing foods (see the "worst" list below) or any alcohol are allowed, and the diet is moderately low-fat.[1,8]

Who should go on the two-week reflux detox in the first place? Obviously, patients who are in the acute decompensated phase must. Those with occasional reflux can benefit from cleaning up their diets by eliminating late-night eating and alcohol rather than following the full-blown detox program. Anyone with reflux who feels they are in the process of decompensating can step back and do a full two-week reflux detox.

Once you have completed the two-week detox program, you cannot just go back to your old habits. Stopping for that slice of pepperoni pizza at midnight after a concert or movie will never again be allowed.

THE REFLUX DETOX DIET: WHAT YOU CAN EAT & DRINK

Agave

Alkaline water

Aloe vera (read label to make sure no vitamin C or acids are added)

Artificial sweetener (maximum of two per day)

Avocados

Bagels and (non-fruit) low-fat muffins

Bananas (great snack food)

Beans (black, red, lima, lentils, etc.)

Bread (especially whole grain and rye)

Caramel (maximum of 4 tablespoons per week)

Celery (great snack food)

Chamomile tea (most other herbal teas are not acceptable)

Chicken (grilled/broiled/baked/steamed without skin)

Chicken stock or bouillon

Coffee (maximum one cup per day, best with milk)

Egg whites

Fennel

Fish (including shellfish, grilled/broiled/baked/steamed)

Ginger (ginger root, ground, or preserved)

Graham crackers

Herbs (excluding all peppers, citrus, garlic, and mustard)

Honey (Manuka honey is preferred)

Melon (honeydew, cantaloupe, watermelon)

Mushrooms (raw or cooked)

Oatmeal (all whole-grain cereals)

Olive oil

Parsley

Popcorn (plain or salted, no butter, no microwave popcorn)

Potatoes (all of the root vegetables are good, except onions)

Rice (especially brown rice, can be a staple during detox)

Skim milk (alternatively, soy or Lactaid skim milk)

Soups (homemade with noodles and low-acid veggies)

Tofu

Turkey breast (no skin)

Vegetables (raw or cooked, but no onions, tomatoes, garlic, or peppers)

Vinaigrette (maximum 1 tablespoon per day, toss salad yourself)

Whole-grain breads, crackers, and breakfast cereals (one serving per day, limit wheat)

Worst and Best Foods for Reflux

All phases of *Dr. Koufman's Acid Reflux Diet* are relatively low-fat and generally exclude "bad fats." You must always limit trans fats, and they are strictly prohibited during the detox program. Meanwhile, olive oil, avocado, and fish all contain "good fat," are rarely associated with reflux, and are allowed.

I can only recall two patients who felt that olive oil caused reflux. Consequently, I no longer limit olive oil, even during the detox. Avocado is an excellent source of good fat, and it does not seem to be associated with reflux either. Listed below are the worst and best foods for reflux.

Worst-for-Reflux Foods and Beverages to Avoid

Onions (a common trigger food that affects some people, not others)

Peppers/hot sauce (all "pepper," including bell and black pepper)

Citrus fruit/juice (these are naturally too acidic for the detox diet)

Fried food (no deep-fried, sautéed in olive oil is permitted)

Fatty meats (beef, bacon, pork, lamb)

Alcoholic beverages (none during detox, and only three per week after that)

Chocolate (one of the worst reflux trigger foods)

All bottled or canned beverages except water (all soft drinks are acidified)

Especially avoid all carbonated beverages (Coke, Pepsi, including seltzer)

Anything that you eat before bed is a "worst for reflux" food.

Bananas (a rich, low-acid fruit, but a trigger food for some people)

Melons (best fruits for most refluxers: watermelon, cantaloupe, honeydew, etc.)

Aloe vera leaf (great thickener and good for digestion, make sure no acid added)

Salads and vegetables (a staple, excluding onions, tomatoes, garlic, and peppers)

Rice and whole grains (best is brown rice, bulgur wheat, whole-grain bread)

Oatmeal (one of the best breakfast foods and great with banana)

Ginger (spicy, zesty flavor but good for reflux—try ginger tea, jam, etc.)

Poultry (baked, grilled, but never fried, skinless preferred, high in protein)

Tofu (coagulated soymilk in many forms, a vegetarian protein)

Fish (all seafood, raw, grilled, baked, broiled, or boiled, and smoked salmon)

This book is primarily intended for people who are on the maintenance phase of the reflux diet. Consequently, in the cookbook section, you will find that there are some recipes that are suitable for the detox phase of the reflux diet and others that are not.

Alkaline Water

Alkaline water is the opposite of acidic and is plentiful, readily available, and can be very helpful in managing reflux because it helps wash out pepsin and is good for pH balancing.[8,31]

Natural alkaline water has trickled through limestone for thousands of years, giving it a pH of between 8.0 and 9.0. Of the brands of alkaline water on the market today, almost half are naturally occurring. Naturally alkaline water is the only potable alkaline substance that is ideal for human consumption, and for reflux sufferers particularly, since there is no other food or beverage that measures above pH 8.0.

We first discovered that alkaline water might be helpful for reflux when some patients reported that drinking alkaline resulted in a "miracle" cure. Even if a person doesn't notice a big improvement in symptoms, alkaline water helps clear pepsin. People who have reflux often have an unhealthy tissue in the respiratory tract and esophagus; drinking acidic beverages further activates the pepsin, whereas alkaline water destroys it.

HERE'S HOW THE pH SCALE WORKS: pH 1.0 to pH 6.9 is acidic, with lower numbers being more acidic. pH 7.0 is neutral (neither acidic nor alkaline). pH 7.1 to 14.0 is alkaline, with the higher numbers being more alkaline. The pH scale, like the earthquake (Richter) scale, is logarithmic, with a difference of one point being 10 times more or less. For example, pH 3.0 is 10 times more acidic than pH 4.0, and pH 2.0 is 100 times more acidic than pH 4.0.

Stomach acid usually has a pH value of between 1.0 and 4.0. The most acidic natural foods we consume are lemons and limes, at about pH 2.6, with all soft drinks falling in that same pH range. The pH value of foods and beverages is not listed on the nutritional label, but if it were, many people would be surprised to see how acidic most popular beverages are.

Using pH monitoring, when we measure the pH in the throat of healthy humans, it is usually about 6.7–6.8. However, with respiratory reflux the average throat pH can be as low as 4.8, which is 100 times more acidic than it should be!

Alkaline water is especially recommended for people who have Barrett's esophagus. The abnormal Barrett's tissue has pepsin in it, and acidic beverages activate the pepsin and cause progression of tissue damage. Alkaline water is recommended as one of the remedies for people with this condition. (See *Beyond Barrett's*, page 82.)

During the two-week reflux detox diet, I recommend drinking only alkaline water. Patients ask if they have to carry alkaline water with them all the time. That is not necessary. There is nothing wrong with drinking ordinary tap water, which is usually about pH 7,[1] but it doesn't kill pepsin.

During transition and even when reflux is in remission, alkaline water is still good for you. Today, most grocery stores, particularly specialty stores, have a large selection of alkaline waters. When you go to the store, look for natural spring water with a pH of 8.0 or higher.

Today, there are special filtration systems and also "alkaline drops" that can be added to ordinary water to make it alkaline. Some of these products work as described and some do not.

Some people just add bicarbonate, or baking soda, to ordinary water to make alkaline water. If you do decide to make your own alkaline water using drops, you should purchase pH paper and test the finished water to be certain that it is in the recommended pH of about 9.0.

CHAPTER 7

Transition Is Trial and Error

Following the two-week reflux detox, most patients report improvement in their symptoms, and on examination, they usually do show improvement. Since most patients start with an RFS of 15 ± 2 at presentation, a post-detox RFS score of 9 demonstrates significant objective improvement.

After detox, I do expect the RFS to be 10 or less (page 35). For patients with coughing and breathing problems—shortness of breath, difficulty taking a full breath in, or asthma-like symptoms—improvement in those symptoms is the first and most important goal.

While these symptoms may not have completely disappeared after detox, there should be improvement. If there isn't, I investigate the possibility that the patient is doing something incorrectly, such as taking acid-suppressive medication after instead of before meals, or the patient is still eating dinner too late. I also review all of the reflux testing data for an explanation for treatment failure. At this point, my treatment algorithm expands, and I may bring other therapeutic options to play. For example, if the patient showed poor esophageal function on manometry, I may prescribe a prokinetic agent, a drug that stimulates (improves) esophageal function.

In rare cases, and depending on all of the data, I recommend a surgical antireflux procedure (see page 45). The point is that treatment failure must be recognized and addressed.

Trigger Foods

When I see improvement, I begin to discuss the transition phase of the reflux diet with the patient. The problem of identifying trigger foods for each individual patient is exemplified by the fact that the banana, a highly recommended food for the reflux diet, is a trigger food for some people.

I recall one woman who had been on therapy for two months, and she was doing relatively well; however, she complained about having mild symptoms every morning after breakfast and at no other time. She reported that her daily breakfast was oatmeal with raisins and a banana. I suggested that she leave off the banana, and her morning symptoms subsequently disappeared. Banana was a trigger food for her.

The purpose of the transition phase is for you to identify your trigger foods. During the detox phase, we prohibit onions, garlic, tomatoes, and peppers (both the vegetables and the seasonings) because all of those are common triggers. In truth, each individual item is a trigger for less than half of people.

After detox, most people want to add all four of those foods back if they can, because they are ingredients in so many different dishes, and for many people they are favorite foods. During transition, our patients add them back in, but one at a time. One person might have trouble with onions and garlic, another with tomatoes and green peppers, and a third might have trouble with just onions.

Of the four items, onions are the most common trigger food, and it appears that some people who have onion as a trigger are very sensitive to it. Even a small amount of onion in a rice dish, for example, might trigger reflux in an onion-sensitive person. Interestingly, cooked onions are generally better (less refluxogenic) than raw onions.

If garlic is a reflux trigger food, it is usually the "meat" of the garlic. Garlic powder and garlic salt are less likely to trigger reflux than the garlic clove itself. For example, sautéing the garlic in oil to get the flavor and then removing it is a successful strategy for some garlic lovers with reflux. (See the garlic-infused olive oil, page 220.)

When it comes to reflux, the tomato is unfairly maligned. As it turns out, fresh tomato is probably a trigger food for fewer than one-third of people. However, because tomato is a very common ingredient in other foods, such as sauces and condiments, it can be inappropriately singled out as the reflux-causing culprit. In other words, as trigger foods go, fresh tomato is different from canned tomato sauce, or even ketchup, both of which are preserved with acids.

Finally, the question of pepper and peppers. Cracked black pepper is a fairly common reflux trigger food. When it comes to bell peppers the vegetable, green peppers appear to be more of a problem than red or yellow ones.

Very few of my patients have sensitivity to all four of these foods. In clinical practice, determining trigger foods for each patient requires adding the foods slowly, and we address dietary questions as they arise, a process that can take months.

We ask some patients to keep a daily food diary to record what they consume and any symptoms that occur as well. If you find that you are uncertain about your triggers, try keeping a food diary for a month.

Trigger foods can cause reflux symptoms immediately, later in the evening, or even the next day. A person might eat a trigger food for dinner and awaken with symptoms the next morning. If you wake up with a sour taste in your mouth, hoarseness, a cough, or a sore throat, you must consider that something that you had for dinner the night before was a trigger. What did you eat that may have caused reflux?

Most of the time, within the context of reflux, the term *trigger* refers to some food or beverage that actually causes reflux. However, the term *trigger* can have other meanings. For example, while cracked pepper may make some patients cough, it's not necessarily that the pepper caused reflux, but rather that the pepper may have stimulated (vagus nerve) cough receptors in the throat. In addition, some trigger foods can cause lightheadedness and sleepiness as well as increases in heart rate and blood pressure. These symptoms also probably occur because of stimulation of vagal nerve receptors in the throat. Finally, anything that burns your mouth or throat when consumed may be a trigger food, too.

One unusual patient reported that when she ate yellowfin tuna, her throat would start burning immediately, and by the time the food was halfway down, she felt that she was refluxing. Yellowfin tuna is an unusual trigger food, but it illustrates the point that any food can be a trigger for someone.

If you have any symptoms after you've eaten something, even the next day, don't ignore it. Figuring out your trigger foods is a kind of sleuthing, and it requires that you pay attention to both your diet and your symptoms.

For the post-detox patient who asks, "So, what can I add back to my diet now?" my first answer is, "What is it that you miss most?" Then, we begin a negotiation. I know the relative risks of different foods based upon my experience with many patients who have been through transition. It is easy to add back foods with the stipulation that it is done systematically.

After detox, we typically allow red apples, pears, berries, condiments, salad dressings, and low-fat cheeses, all in small amounts. However, when eating out, you must always add your own condiments, salad dressings, sauces, and cheeses yourself—that is, ask for them on the side. You will usually add less than the kitchen will.

We also allow more coffee and tea, as well as lean pork and yogurt. The least acidic yogurt brands are listed in a post on www.refluxcookbook-blog.com. For meat lovers, we allow lean beef twice a month, but still prohibit fatty beef, lamb, and bacon.

Most Common Reflux Trigger Foods

Chocolate
High-fat meats
Deep-fried food
Alcohol
Nuts
Coffee
Onions
Tomatoes
Apples
Garlic
Strawberries
Cracked pepper
Bell peppers (green worse than red)
Bread (for some, gluten may be a trigger)

A discussion of trigger foods would not be complete without discussing the rare, difficult-to-solve case. Some trigger foods are hard to pin down. For example, one patient's reflux was under reasonably good control—she was off medication and was usually asymptomatic—but some mornings she still awoke with reflux symptoms.

She was not a regular wine drinker, but as it turns out, she was very sensitive to white wine. When she was out she would sometimes accept a glass of white wine even though she had no intention of drinking the entire glass. Someone might propose a toast, and glasses were raised, and she would take a few small sips. It took a while to figure out that she was very sensitive to white wine, which was a trigger for her.

Here are some examples of the trigger-food profiles of three of my patients:

Patient #1: chocolate, coffee, onions, garlic, cucumbers, white wine, cashews, macadamia nuts, green peppers, red delicious apples, and cheese

Patient #2: chocolate, green peppers, black pepper, and alcohol

Patient #3: onions, most nuts, and alcohol

Remember, as you go forward, stay away from high-fat, high-caffeine, high-risk-for-trigger foods until you are certain that your reflux is in good shape. Even after you have started eating healthier and you are getting over your reflux, you will still be vulnerable to indiscretions for a few months. Proceed slowly.

In the end, trigger-food identification is the hardest part about beating reflux. You will identify your triggers soon enough, but the bigger questions will be the time at which you eat dinner, how you handle social engagements, how much alcohol you drink, and whether you can live without processed food, fast food, or junk food.

Several years ago, we allowed our reflux patients to eat unrestricted amounts of bread, but we now believe that bread (i.e., gluten) is a reflux trigger for some people who do not have celiac disease. The gluten in bread causes some people to reflux, but as of this writing, the mechanism and magnitude of this problem remain unknown. (See *Pick Your Poison or Cure,* page 75.)

Water, Water, Everywhere and Nothing Left to Drink

Even if it says "healthy" on the label, almost every drink in a bottle or can is like poison. If this seems like a bold statement, consider that (excluding still water) almost everything bottled and canned has the same acidity as stomach acid, and contains chemicals that have been shown to be harmful, if not cancer-causing, as well as artificial sweeteners that have their own recently discovered toxic profiles.

Water, and ideally alkaline water, is the best thing you can drink day in and day out.[31] To that, you may add coffee and tea that is not prepackaged. Incidentally, coffee is less of a reflux trigger than people think. It is a trigger for only about 25 percent of reflux sufferers. For most people, several cups of coffee a day are fine after detox. However, if you consume a pot of coffee before noon, the caffeine itself will cause reflux, because caffeine makes the lower esophageal sphincter relax.

People who are sensitive to coffee as a reflux trigger tend to be *very* sensitive to it, and even small amounts—decaf or caffeinated—can trigger reflux. For coffee-sensitive individuals who want a little caffeine to get started in the morning, black or green tea is a good substitute.

So what else can you drink? Soft drinks are gone, of course, and that is permanent. Can you ever have a glass of orange juice? The answer is yes, but there is a big difference between having a glass of orange juice with brunch on Sunday and drinking half a gallon of the stuff every day.

Now comes the question you've been waiting for—what about alcohol? There is no getting around it: Alcohol and reflux are intimately intertwined. Alcohol is a huge cause of reflux, and in my practice, the patients who have the most trouble beating reflux are alcoholics. Alcohol is up there at the top of the reflux trigger list, along with chocolate and fried food, and taking an acid-suppressive medication like a PPI does not give you permission to consume alcohol.

I also do have patients who like a glass of wine with dinner, and for many people, a glass of wine does not cause trouble. However, two glasses of wine, or wine consumed after 8 p.m. may very well be associated with reflux.

pH Balancing

When patients come off the two-week detox program and they want to reintroduce fruit with more acidity than melons and bananas, pH balancing becomes important. For example, if berries are added to cereal with soy, almond, or cow's milk—all of which are alkaline—then pH balancing is automatically achieved.

Acidic fruit alone can be followed with alkaline water as a chaser. pH balancing is basic: consume acidic foods with alkaline foods. Here are a few other examples of pH balancing: coffee with milk, fruit jelly on bread, and turkey burgers with dill pickles.

One of the most common food questions I am asked is about lemons and limes. In the past, I would have said that those are absolutely prohibited, but that is no longer the case. Using lemon or lime in small amounts as a flavoring is probably not going to cause problems for most people after reflux is under control. They should be used sparingly and preferably with alkaline water with the meal. Meanwhile, if you consume lemon or lime and this causes symptoms, particularly throat burning, you must avoid them. Zest, or the peel of the lemon or lime, is not acidic. It is the fruit and juice inside that is acidic.

In some of the recipes in this book you'll see acidic ingredients, but rest assured that every recipe is pH balanced—none are acidic. To learn more about the foods and beverages that are most alkaline, see *Dropping Acid: The Reflux Diet Cookbook & Cure* and its companion website, www.refluxcookbookblog.com.

CHAPTER 8

Maintenance Phase

When I was young, someone told me that 20 percent of life is spent on maintenance. At the time I bristled at the idea. I was too busy for that.

As I have grown older, I find that I spend a lot more time maintaining everything, not the least of which is my dietary health. I cook most of my own food now, and I plan time for exercise and relaxation. It is my goal to convince you, even if you are still young, that health maintenance and disease prevention are essential, and it starts with what and when you eat.

I think of reflux maintenance as the stage when good, long-term habits are formed. The habits that are important in maintaining health involve aspects that are not specifically diet-related. For example, if you have reflux and your spouse gets home from work at 8:30 in the evening, then dinner together may be a problem. Negotiations have to take place between partners to reach consensus, a way of managing meals that works for you both.

You may also have to change your work schedule and your social life. A psychotherapist who works until 9:00 p.m., for example, might have to take a break from 5:00 to 6:00 for dinner.

You will need to take your work situation and family responsibilities into consideration. In my practice, the biggest fight my patients face is over dinnertime, specifically the time the patient can arrive home, prepare dinner, and eat. Dinner at 6:00 p.m. is no doubt one of the biggest adjustments for most people. Dinner should be your special meal, but it should not be the meal when you refuel for the day. You should try to obtain 75 percent of your calories each day before 5:00 p.m.

> It is important to emphasize that late-night eating is the single most important risk factor for many refluxers. It probably does not matter how "healthy" you eat if you're eating it late.

I have had many patients whose reflux remained recalcitrant until they were able to move dinner to an early hour. In addition, lying down right after dinner and late nights of heavy drinking are incompatible with reflux health.

The maintenance phase involves planning meals, cooking, bringing food to work, and training friends and family. You must establish routines for meals, snacks, and even dining out. Introduce your dietary needs to the server at restaurants: "Hi, I am on a special diet. I would like to know what grilled fish or fowl is available that does not have butter or sauce on it—olive oil is fine."

In order to achieve and continue maintenance, you must have a plan. You should have a variety of go-to meals. You should have at least three breakfasts that can be ordered from a restaurant and three breakfasts that can be made at home. Depending upon your work, you may have to bring lunch and daytime snacks with you. Figure out which lunch options work best for you and then make sure that you have a cooler and/or refrigerator to store your food. You will need proper food containers for transporting food. I double-bag; I have found self-closing plastic bags to be excellent for most foods, especially when smaller bags are placed within a one-gallon bag to prevent spillage.

You will have to cook, or at the very least prepare, some food. Options that work on-the-go include hard-boiled eggs, turkey burgers, chicken breasts, rice, fruit, smoothies, and salads. Make a list of all the snacks you like that fit within the reflux guidelines.

Pick your days for shopping and food preparation. I recommend that you have a standard cooking time set aside twice a week, plus at least one on the weekend. Personally, I shoot for Thursday and Monday evenings when I can cook at my leisure. Create a shopping list on your computer that's easy to handle as a checklist. It is going to be important for you to keep staples that you like in your kitchen.

Part of maintenance is planning so that you have enough to eat. That said, every meal need not be a delight. On those days when I am faced with a demanding schedule, two hard-boiled eggs suffice for breakfast, a banana is the morning snack, and leftover soup or fish and rice are my lunch.

Learn to eat new things. Many of the recipes contained in this book are easily transported and can be used for additional meals during the week.

Planning, Cooking, and Meal Plans

On the pages that follow, you will find the one-week meal plan template and three meal plans. Using the template to create your own meal plan is best. Try not to eat the same foods week after week. You should modify your diet periodically based on new discoveries, especially new recipes and new foods.

I discovered that I love the Roasted Cauliflower & Watercress Miso Chowder (page 120) for dinner and cold the next day for lunch. I also love the Gluten-Free Pumpkin Muffins (page 97), both in the morning for breakfast and as a sweet snack or dessert.

Planning and cooking are necessary if you are going to keep to *Dr. Koufman's Acid Reflux Diet*. Think discipline and structure, but think fun and adventure as well. Creation of a meal plan a week ahead is—well—basic planning.

Before you start, there are several key variables: home-cooked vs. store-bought, and home or workplace eating vs. dining out. Store-bought means takeout from a restaurant, bodega, or grocery store. So you can cook it or have it cooked for you, *and* you can eat it at home or away from home.

> **To get the best results, you should make your own meal plan; the process of planning what you will do for the week ahead is key.**

Now, each day, I recommend that you have three meals and two snacks, so to cover the workweek (Monday through Friday) plus the weekend (Saturday and Sunday), you will have to fill in 35 boxes.

Here is the sequence that I recommend to fill out your meal plan for the week:

1. Fill in all eating-out dates and restaurants first. This includes breakfast, lunch, and dinner engagements, even coffee or "high tea."

2. Decide which days you will cook (designated "Cooking Days") and prepare food and/or shop. Obviously, you can shop another day in advance if you like.

3. Before you fill out the meal plan, fill out the B, S, L, D lines: B1, B2, B3 are three breakfasts; L1, L2, L3 are three lunches; D1, D2, D3 are three dinners; and S1, S2, S3 are three snacks. You can write in more, for example, B4, S4, L4, etc.

4. With each, determine where it will come from: BFH (brought from home), TO (takeout), etc.

5. Create a shopping list for the foods that you will need for cooking, as well as other brought-from-home items such as alkaline water, fruits, etc.

6. Fill out the 14 snacks for the week first, and remember that if you need food at work, you are going to have to bring it. If you have a refrigerator at work, that's great; if not, you will need a good-quality cooler.

7. Finally, fill out the entire meal-plan grid, and then check to see if your shopping list matches your food requirements.

On the pages that follow, you will find the one-week meal plan template and three sample meal plans, one by each author. They are provided to demonstrate the different ways people eat. My meal plan is pretty close to the detox diet. Sonia and Chef Philip cook most of their own meals.

MEAL PLAN FOR_____

NAME

	MONDAY	TUESDAY	WEDNESDAY
BREAKFAST			
SNACK			
LUNCH			
SNACK			
DINNER			

Weekly meal plan should have 3 breakfast (B), 3 lunch (L), and 3 snack (S), and 3 dinner (D) choices

B1 _____   S1 _____   L1 _____

B2 _____   S2 _____   L2 _____

B3 _____   S3 _____   L3 _____

Shop/Cook Day 1 _____ | _____

Shop/Cook Day 2 _____ | _____

Shop/Cook Day 3 _____ | _____

Dr. Koufman's Acid Reflux Diet

THE WEEK OF _____

THURSDAY	FRIDAY	SATURDAY	SUNDAY

D1 _____

D2 _____

D3 _____

H Home
W Work
R Restaurant
O Other (like at a friend's place)
TO Takeout
C Cooked by you at home
GS Grocery Store
BFH Brought from home

_____

_____

_____

MEAL PLAN FOR _____ **Dr. Jamie** _____

	MONDAY	TUESDAY	WEDNESDAY
BREAKFAST	W TO Lox omelet	W BFH Salmon & rice leftovers	W TO Lox omelet
SNACK	W BFH Banana	W BFH Pumpkin muffin	W BFH Avocado
LUNCH	W TO Chicken & veggies	W TO Sushi	W TO Shrimp & salad
SNACK	W BFH Avocado	W BFH Banana	W BFH Pumpkin muffin
DINNER	H C Salmon; rice; veggies; Pumpkin muffin	R 5.45pm Hangawi with Roger	R 5.45pm Momoya with Dora

Weekly meal plan should have 3 breakfast (B), 3 lunch (L), and 3 snack (S), and 3 dinner (D) choices

B1 Omelet (p 103)   S1 Banana   L1 Chicken & Veggies

B2 Smoothie (p 100)   S2 Pumpkin muffin (p 97)   L2 Shrimp & Salad

B3 Frittata (p 95)   S3 Royal eggs (p 198)   L3 Shrimp & Zucchini (p 185)

Shop/Cook Day 1 _____ | I usually cook and shop Sunday, Monday, and Thursday. _____

Shop/Cook Day 2 _____ | _____

Shop/Cook Day 3 _____ | _____

THURSDAY	FRIDAY	SATURDAY	SUNDAY
H ························· C Smoothie	W ························· TO Lox omelet	H ························· C Smoothie	H ························· C Frittata; fruit; coffee
W ························· BFH Pumpkin muffin	W ························· BFH Royal eggs	W ························· BFH Avocado	
W ························· TO Chicken & veggies	W ························· C Turkey burger	R ························· 6p Restaurant Loi with Edythe	H ························· C Shrimp & zucchini pasta; rice; veggies
W ························· BFH Avocado	W ························· BFH Avocado	H ························· GS Banana	H ························· GS Banana
H ························· C Cauliflower chowder; salad	R ················ 5.45pm Restaurant Daniel with Erika	O ················· 6pm Dinner at Ricky's	H ························· C Turkey Burger Salad

H Home
W Work
R Restaurant
O Other (like at a friend's place)
TO Takeout
C Cooked by you at home
GS Grocery Store
BFH Brought from home

D1 Salmon (p 147), Rice (p 151)

D2 Cauliflower Chowder (p 120)

D3 Turkey Burger Salad (p 185)

BTW: My diet is almost always close to the reflux detox diet.

_____

_____

MEAL PLAN FOR _____ **Sonia**

	MONDAY	TUESDAY	WEDNESDAY
BREAKFAST	W　　　　　　TO Egg white omelet; coffee	W　　　　　　TO Egg white omelet; coffee	H　　　　　　C Smoothie; coffee
SNACK	W　　　　　BFH Melon slices	W　　　　　BFH Banana	W　　　　　BFH Carrot sticks & hummus
LUNCH	W　　　　　BFH Cauliflower Miso Chowder; rice crackers	W　　　　　BFH Shrimp & Tofu Soup; salad	W　　　　　BFH Cold Somen Noodles with Dipping Sauce; veggies
SNACK	W　　　　　BFH Popcorn with Rosemary & Salt	W　　　　　BFH Pumpkin muffin	W　　　　　BFH Low-fat cheddar cheese with rice crackers
DINNER	H　　　　　　C Linguine with Mussels & Arugula; salad	H　　　　　　C One-Pot Chicken; Stir-fried Green Beans	H　　　　　　C Shrimp & Peas; rice; Corn with Miso & Basil

NOTE: I shop for and make different meals daily for variety.

B1 Omelet (p 102)　　　　　S1 Popcorn (p 109)　　　　　L1 Cauliflower Chowder (p 120)

B2 Smoothie (p 100)　　　　S2 Muffin (p 97 or 98)　　　　L2 Somen Noodles (p 104)

B3 Rice Porridge (p 105)　　S3 Marbled Tea Eggs (p 197)　L3 Cold Noodles (p 158)

B4 Frittata (p 95)　　　　　S4 Pearl Balls (p 196)　　　　L4 Pickled Bean Sprouts (p 160)

B5 _____　　　　S5 Lettuce Cups (p 202)　　　　L5 Basil Chicken (p 176)

B6 _____　　　　S6 _____　　　　L6 Jade Fried Rice (p 153)

THURSDAY	FRIDAY	SATURDAY	SUNDAY
W　　　　　　TO Egg white omelet; coffee	H　　　　　　C Bagel; fruit; coffee	H　　　　　　C Rice Porridge with Chicken; veggies; coffee	H　　　　　　C Supa-Dupa Vegan Frittata; fruit; coffee
W　　　　　BFH Caramel Apple Muffin	W　　　　　BFH Marbled Tea Eggs	H　　　　　GS Fuji apple	H　　　　　GS Graham crackers
W　　　　　BFH Salmon fried rice; steamed veggies	W　　　　　BFH Cold Noodles with Sesame Sauce; veggies	H　　　　　C Pickled Bean Sprouts; Basil Chicken; rice	H　　　　　C Emperor's Jade Fried Rice; Green Beans
W　　　　　BFH Carrot sticks & hummus	W　　　　　BFH Banana	H　　　　　C Pearl Balls; sliced cucumbers	H　　　　　C Lettuce Cups with Pine Nuts
H　　　　　C Tempeh Marsala; Stir-fried Brussels Sprouts	R　　　　6pm Dinner with Christopher at Nobu	H　　　　　C Tofu Cutlet; Spinach with sesame dressing	H　　　　　C Poached Halibut; Rice; Taiwanese Dill with GInger

D1 <u>Linguine with Mussels & Arugula (p 192)</u>

D2 <u>One-Pot Chicken (p 170), Stir-fried Green Beans (p 157)</u>

D3 <u>Stir-fried Shrimp & Peas (p 190), Stir-fried Corn (p 159)</u>

D4 <u>Tempeh Marsala (p 174), Stir-fried Brussels Sprouts (p 150)</u>

D5 <u>Tofu Cutlet (p 175)</u>

D6 <u>Poached Halibut with Prosciutto (p 177), Taiwanese Dill (p 161)</u>

H Home
W Work
R Restaurant
O Other (like at a friend's place)
TO Takeout
C Cooked by you at home
GS Grocery Store
BFH Brought from home

MEAL PLAN FOR_____ **Chef Philip**_____

	MONDAY	TUESDAY	WEDNESDAY
BREAKFAST	H C Bagel	H C Smoothie	H C Tea and pastry
SNACK			
LUNCH	H C Burrito	H C Orange tofu with broccoli and rice	H C Vegan pizza
SNACK			
DINNER	H C Paella	H C Risotto with tempeh cutlets and greens	H C Vegetable hot pot

Weekly meal plan should have 3 breakfast (B), 3 lunch (L), and 3 snack (S), and 3 dinner (D) choices

B1 _____   S1 _____   L1 _____

B2 _____   S2 _____   L2 _____

B3 _____   S3 _____   L3 _____

Shop/Cook Day 1 _____ | I cook every day and I don't snack._____

Shop/Cook Day 2 _____ | _____

Shop/Cook Day 3 _____ | _____

Typical Week

THURSDAY	FRIDAY	SATURDAY	SUNDAY
H C Smoothie	H C Fresh fruit	H C Tofu scramble with potatoes	Nothing (sleep in)
H C Veggie burger with baked potato	H C Burrito	H C Salad with grilled peppers and potatoes	H C Black beans and rice
R 6pm Ethiopian Restaurant	H C Cold noodles with cucumbers and soybeans	H C Turned cornmeal with sautéed okra	H C Grilled tempeh; sautéed collards

D1 _____

D2 _____

D3 _____

H Home
W Work
R Restaurant
O Other (like at a friend's place)
TO Takeout
C Cooked by you at home
GS Grocery Store
BFH Brought from home

Dining Out

Depending upon your stage of the reflux diet, you will have different degrees of freedom when dining out. If you are on the two-week reflux detox diet, you will have to go to a restaurant that serves grilled, baked, or broiled fish or chicken, a salad with no dressing, and grilled vegetables. There is no butter, cheese, or sauce during detox.

During the transition, maintenance, and longevity phases, planning is still necessary, but it gets easier as you gain experience and health. In general, ethnic restaurants (e.g., Mexican, Italian, Chinese) make it harder, but not impossible, to maintain your reflux diet.

If you are on a really limited diet, you're going to have to think about where to eat out and what you can order before you go. Most restaurants have their menus online, so it is easy to see your options, even if you've never eaten there before. This awareness means communicating with friends, relatives, and business associates before dinner reservations are made. Tell your fellow diners in advance, "I am on a restricted diet, and I would prefer it if we could dine at a ____ restaurant (fill in the blank), and how about a 6:00 p.m. reservation?"

Furthermore, if you are on an especially restricted diet—gluten-free and dairy-free, for example—you have to negotiate with your server when ordering. You must specify that you do not eat butter, cheese, bread, or pasta (unless it is gluten-free), and you must ask how the fish/chicken/beef is prepared.

> **In an Italian restaurant, the grilled octopus and the branzino (sometimes listed on the menu as Mediterranean sea bass), prepared in olive oil (not corn oil or butter), are excellent menu choices.**

I am gluten-free, dairy-free, and sugar-free, and one of my favorite restaurants in New York is a well-known French restaurant. On my first visit, I explained my diet. I was surprised when the response was, "No problem . . . no problem, except for desserts." They would bring me an appetizer and sympathetically announce, "Instead of *crème fraîche* on your shrimp, there is a *confit* of melons." As time passed, I became friendly with the servers and the chef so that when I went to the restaurant, the server would ask with a smile, "So, Doctor Koufman, are you still not eating desserts?" That was their code to let me know that they still understood the limitations of my diet and could still accommodate them.

> It makes sense to begin creating consensus and familiarity among friends and co-workers, chefs and restaurants, about how you eat. It gets easier over time.

The key variables to successful restaurant dining are the front-end negotiations with your dining companions and with the restaurant staff. If you are shy and think special orders can be disruptive, consider that, today, almost half of people dining in restaurants have some kind of special order. Things have changed, and servers and restaurants are now used to accommodating "fussy" eaters. Get to know the staff, and you will find better choices, food, and service. And the upside is that you will establish a repertoire of suitable, maybe even terrific, restaurants that know you and will cater to you.

It is also important to keep people accountable. If you are gluten-free, for example, and you get sick after dining in a restaurant, call the restaurant and complain. Think of yourself as a consumer who cares about what you are consuming. If you took your car to a car wash and it was still dirty afterward, wouldn't you say something? If you are a good consumer, act like one, especially when it comes to your food.

Again comes the question of what to drink. Water, coffee, and iced tea are your best basic choices. A discussion of alcohol as a trigger food can be found on page 58.

Now we return to the tricky part. Almost everything we have discussed so far might not rigidly apply to you. If you are in the maintenance and longevity phases of the diet, you are no longer really a refluxer, are you? You are in remission. So, the question becomes, how much can you cheat, and is it really cheating? Yes, you should probably continue to avoid your big trigger foods, as well as all bottled and canned beverages excluding water. However, "reflux-unfriendly" foods may be fine on occasion. As you will see in the recipe section, we sometimes use wine and vinegar and sesame oil, all potential trigger foods for some people, but not for most. This is one of the areas of reflux management that you must do for yourself—that is, identify your trigger foods (see page 53).

When you are healthy, you do not need to color within the lines all the time. The basics don't change, but the details can. The key is to know your limits and avoid making unnecessary and costly mistakes. As you change how you eat and plan your meals, you will also change how you think about food. As you mature as a healthy eater, you will find that dining out is pleasurable and easy despite the fact that you order with care.

CHAPTER 9

The Longevity Diet

After months or years of living a healthy lifestyle, you don't have to think about what you can eat anymore. It is automatic. When you know that fruits, vegetables, and other foods vary by season and location, you simply pick the best variety. But, planning is always necessary—for example, you may always need to prepare and bring food to your workplace.

This stage of *Dr. Koufman's Acid Reflux Diet* is called the longevity diet because we believe that if you follow this diet, you will live to a healthy old age. About half the nation says that they are interested in changing how they eat, and this is the healthy half.

Here's the startling paradigm shift for the other half—food is fuel for your body, and it should never have become an all-consuming, all-day, every day obsession. Furthermore, the food industry, through marketing and political influence, has made it hard to eat real food and hard to avoid food that isn't good for us. That might in part explain why there are so many different dietary factions today: omnivorous, vegetarian, vegan, pescatarian, gluten-free, sugar-free, dairy-free, chemical-free, and so on.

Pick Your Poison or Cure

Omnivores may eat everything that is animal- or plant-derived. The difference between vegan and vegetarian is that a vegan won't consume any animal products. Some vegans also try to eliminate all animal products from their lives, including things like leather and wool. Vegetarians do not eat meat, fish, or poultry, but they may eat eggs and dairy products, including yogurt, milk, and cheese. Pescatarians are fish eaters but not meat eaters; they may otherwise be vegetarian. There are thousands of possible combinations, and you must decide for yourself what choices you make. Even if you are an omnivore, you still may want to limit red meat, both because of the risk of reflux and because the fat is unhealthy fat.

The concept of a longevity diet, particularly *your* longevity diet, must take into account everything from your family history of heart disease and diabetes, to autoimmune diseases, your weight, your reflux trigger foods, your ethnicity, and your dietary preferences. If you have food sensitivities, such as gluten and dairy, those will have to be taken into consideration as well.

The question of what constitutes a healthy diet, a longevity diet, is changing, and I like to think that we now know more than ever before. It's true that if you read enough about food and health, almost nothing you eat appears to be completely safe and healthy. That said, the thrust of this book and the recipes is *lean, clean, green,* and *alkaline.* If you add in food sensitivities and take away trigger foods, there may be a limited number of foods and recipes that will fully satisfy your situation. That's life.

Most of our recipes are vegan and gluten-free because that's who we are, and because those are the recipes most requested by our patients. The real debate, dilemma, and hard part for you is probably going to be about sugar.

Bread and Sugar Addiction

Our first book emphasized that acid was bad for reflux, and we recommended eating a lot of bread, but we now know more about bread.[2,4] As attention to gluten, sugar, and bread in relationship to obesity have gained prominence in the media, there has been a big shift. While some people think that being gluten-free is a fad—as of this writing, approximately 30 percent of the American population identifies as gluten-free—the issue is here to stay, and it is complicated by changes in bread—in the hybridized wheat with which most bread is made today.[2]

In 1970, Norman Borlaug won the Nobel Peace Prize for inventing a new form of hybridized wheat that people thought would end world hunger. Borlaug's wheat is disease- and drought-resistant and increases yields tenfold per acre.[2] Unfortunately, the image of amber waves of grain swaying in the wind must be replaced by the image of "dwarf wheat" with large popcorn-like kernels of gluten attached. This is not the wheat that our parents grew up eating. One big difference is its sugar content. The gylcemic (sugar conversion) index of cane sugar, the stuff in your sugar bowl, is 59. The glycemic index of bread made with Borlaug's dwarf wheat is 72.[2] Today, bread products made with this genetically altered wheat is about all you can get.

The sugar in the bread that we eat with breakfast, lunch, dinner, and snacks must be added to the sugar that is loaded into other food products we consume. This amounts to a great deal of sugar. Sugar addiction and alcohol addiction probably share more similarities than most people might think, but I believe that sugar is even more addictive than alcohol, because the more sugar you eat, the more you want.[3]

Breaking your sugar addiction may be the hardest thing you've ever done. Nevertheless, many of my patients have been able to do it. The unfortunate truth is that if you are obese, you are almost certainly addicted to sugar. The program that I recommend below is not the only way to go— many people just try to cut back, and do so successfully. Maybe giving up sweets and limiting bread can work for you. I suspect that there may be as many ways to cut sugar from one's diet as there are individuals who want to do it.

Notably, not all sugar is created equal, and fructose, as in *high-fructose corn syrup* (HFCS), is more harmful than other sugars.[3] Nevertheless, all carbohydrates should be considered sugar. As you will see below, the idea is to get natural sugars from natural foods, rather than HFCS, which is in many processed products, including breakfast cereals, muffins, crackers, soups, salad dressings, and condiments.

You may substitute one sugar for another at the beginning and slowly try to reduce your intake of sugar and carbs over time. One serving of fruit and one serving of potato or rice per day is plenty.

SEVEN STEPS FOR QUITTING (OR REDUCING) SUGAR

1. Get high-fructose corn syrup out of your diet. Also, abstain from bread, pasta, cookies, cakes, energy bars, doughnuts, and everything else you know that contains added sugar. And yes, you really do have to quit bread, at least at the beginning.

2. When you crave bread, think fruit. During the first few weeks of bread and sugar abstinence, your sugar craving can be satisfied by fruits such as figs, dates, bananas, and red apples. Organic dates are loaded with sugar, and I suspect that three of them are roughly equivalent to the sugar content of a candy bar. It's okay if you eat more than three at the beginning, but later on you will want to reduce the sugar, with just one or two for a snack or dessert.

3. Stop eating sugary breakfast cereals and substitute gluten-free oatmeal with raisins and banana, or other breakfast items that are sugar-free. The Everyday Lox Omelet (page 103) is an example of an excellent alternative breakfast that you can make at home or get in a restaurant.

4. If you are still drinking soft drinks, stop! Drink water, and drink coffee and tea in moderation. If you are going to drink iced tea, make it yourself and do not use an artificial sweetener; get used to drinking it plain.

5. You can satisfy your craving for carbohydrates with potatoes, rice, and gluten-free and sugar-free chips or crackers. Read labels to make sure that there are no trans fats in any of these items. Sweet potatoes and baked potatoes are an excellent carb alternative to sugar. Baked potatoes are best when consumed with olive oil rather than butter or sour cream.

6. Begin to scrutinize the nutritional information on all of the products that you consider staples in your home. Chicken stock, for example, usually has sugar added. Make your own (see page 217), or look for a brand that has no sugar and stockpile it so you have as much as you need for day-to-day cooking, especially if you use chicken stock in many recipes. You also will find that many condiments have sugar

added. Unfortunately, for both its acidity and its added sugar, you should consider eliminating ketchup from your diet.

7. Finally, begin to reduce your overall reliance on carbohydrates, including complex carbohydrates. You will find that your body prefers protein and good fats and that eggs, poultry, fish, avocado, olive oil, rice, tofu, vegetables, and salads will become go-to foods. If you need a dessert after a meal, make it fruit.

> **If you are going to really eat healthy, quickly clean out your house; get rid of the cookies, snack foods, ice cream, and all of the other overly acidic, sugary, and prohibited foods.**

In case it isn't already clear: when you quit gluten, you must quit sugar as well, because almost all gluten-free bread, cookies, etc., are loaded with sugar and should be avoided. And why go dairy-free as well? Unless dairy is restricted, overeaters and obese people will gravitate toward consumption of high-fat dairy products such as cheese and ice cream. What does this leave? A lean diet that is mostly fish, fowl, fruits, vegetables, and non-gluten grains.

There is no specific time period for how long it will take you to be free of processed sugar, but if you are going to break sugar addiction, you have to view it as an addiction.

Carbohydrate Intolerance

Some of my "recovered" sugar addicts subsequently develop carbohydrate intolerance. Usually, this happens to patients who had been gluten-free and sugar-free for months or years. After consuming carbohydrates, their blood pressure and pulse rate increase, and within minutes, they experience sinking fatigue. Eating dates might make such a person drowsy to the point of falling asleep. For some, the carbohydrate intolerance is progressive, so over time more symptoms appear with smaller carbohydrate loads. Eating figs, which are naturally high in sugar, might be expected to cause symptoms, but as time passes, such patients may even develop difficulty in tolerating modest amounts of rice or potato.

In addition, some of these patients report toe, foot, and leg cramps hours after eating carbohydrates, and some report that their urine smells sweet. The foot/leg cramps usually occur in the evening and can be severe enough to wake a person from a sound sleep. The mechanism of these sugar-caused cramps is unknown. The sweet-smelling urine suggests that there is sugar in the urine. While this is usually seen in diabetics, we are finding this phenomenon in our post-sugar-addiction, carbohydrate-resistant patients who don't have diabetes. This suggests that their bodies no longer have the metabolic machinery to handle a sugar load.

The medical literature on carbohydrate intolerance doesn't address this syndrome; it suggests that carbohydrate intolerance is related to gluten sensitivity and diabetes. This is not the case in my experience. The syndrome that I have observed is different. I believe that carbohydrate intolerance may be related to a still-unknown mechanism associated with sugar metabolism.

Imagine that the super sugar-addicted person revs up all the hormones and cellular metabolic equipment that deal with sugar. Now, imagine quitting sugar. What if those metabolic factories just shut down like a ghost town after a key industry has moved away? I do not have the answer, but the problems of sugar addiction and "rebound" carbohydrate intolerance that go beyond the risk of diabetes deserve further investigation.

This brings me to the question of actual gluten sensitivity. I first became aware of the problem years ago when a patient with reflux told me that she was gluten-sensitive. She asked if I had a list of foods that were safe for reflux and were gluten-free. I didn't. Furthermore, that first gluten-sensitive patient forced me to think about the question of bread, pasta, and many of the products that were on our good-for-reflux list.

Not long after, a young and otherwise healthy patient who had been resistant to reflux treatment for a year came in with a dramatic improvement, and she announced that she had conquered her reflux by going gluten-free. Since that time, I have found many reflux patients for whom a gluten-free diet has been the difference in outcome. Though still difficult to estimate, I suspect that the problem of gluten sensitivity is bigger than celiac disease and gluten-associated reflux.

Earlier in this book, I noted that I am gluten-free, sugar-free, and dairy-free. I share my story here because I believe that my condition is another manifestation of gluten sensitivity about which the medical establishment does not yet know much.

Two years ago, after complaining to my doctor that my psoriasis was out of control and that my balance was poor, she confirmed that my cerebellar (balance) testing was abnormal. I underwent a brain scan to make sure that I didn't have a brain tumor, which I did not. I was tested for food sensitivities and was found to have sensitivities to gluten (and milk).

My diagnosis was gluten ataxia, which is a condition in which the target organ for gluten sensitivity is the brain, particularly the cerebellum.[46,47] Since that time, I have strictly avoided gluten, and my overall health has improved, including my balance and my psoriasis.[48]

Psoriasis, rheumatoid arthritis, Hashimoto's thyroiditis, and certain kidney diseases are believed to be autoimmune diseases. When I went to medical school, we thought that autoimmunity was the result of a prior viral infection. The idea was that when your body made antibodies to the virus—some part of you having similar proteins as those in the virus— the antibodies subsequently attacked that part of you. Today, we are beginning to think about autoimmunity differently. For years, I've listened to my patients as they shared personal stories about their own diseases and their own cures. It now seems likely that food sensitivities play a much larger role than previously thought in many common diseases. As sophisticated diagnostic testing becomes more available and affordable, I suspect that the science of food sensitivity will expand dramatically and result in new ways of treating the root causes of many autoimmune diseases like gluten ataxia.

It was my intention for this book to be a cookbook first and a medical book second. It is inevitable, however, that I feel compelled to address questions about nutrition and diet that affect my patients and that are still on the cutting edge of science. Clearly, the medical mainstream does not yet understand that many diseases can be reversed and/or prevented through diet.

I also suspect that for many readers, this book, and particularly this section, will raise more questions than it answers. If that is the case for you,

I am pleased. I would like for you to think of this book as a starting point toward a new understanding of nutrition and health—in particular, how food affects *you*.

So what to eat? All the choices—vegetarian, vegan, pescatarian, gluten-free, sugar-free, dairy-free—are yours. Pick your poison or cure.

Beyond Barrett's

Before the publication of *Dropping Acid: The Reflux Diet Cookbook & Cure*, my practice consisted mostly of people with respiratory reflux and voice disorders. After the book's publication, my office was filled with patients suffering from every manifestation of reflux, including patients with Barrett's esophagus, a condition caused by years of esophageal reflux.[32,34,49]

For some of my Barrett's patients, the diagnosis was unexpected. The typical story: A patient was scheduled to have a colonoscopy, and the gastroenterologist suggested that he undergo an upper endoscopy (esophagogastroduodenoscopy, or EGD) at the same time. A week later, the patient receives a telephone call, "Your biopsies showed Barrett's esophagus." He received a prescription for a PPI and was told to come back for a repeat endoscopy in a year. That was the extent of his medical advice. So, as many do, the upset patient turned to the Internet and discovered that Barrett's is precancerous and that esophageal cancer is deadly. Terrified, the patient searched for more information and found me.

Most of the Barrett's patients who come to me are desperate and afraid, and in no small measure this book was written for my Barrett's patients who asked, "If I always eat healthy and alkaline, can I prevent esophageal cancer?" The answer is YES! Barrett's doesn't cause cancer, reflux does. As a matter of fact, Barrett's is not supposed to be reversible, but it is.

A patient from Seattle came to see me a year after she had been diagnosed with Barrett's. She had been enrolled in the Seattle Barrett's Esophagus Project after having been positively diagnosed by biopsy. After she read *Dropping Acid: The Reflux Diet Cookbook & Cure,* she put herself on the strict reflux detox diet for a full year. At that point, she came to see me and asked that I perform a transnasal esophagoscopy (TNE) on her. I did, and her Barrett's was gone—reversed with a low-acid diet and alkaline water![32]

Before discussing how my reflux diet might be modified for people with Barrett's esophagus, permit me to share some additional thoughts about Barrett's.

In the past, it was believed that people with Barrett's had a one-percent chance per year of getting esophageal cancer. It is now clear that that estimate is far too high and that progression from Barrett's to esophageal cancer is uncommon. It is particularly uncommon in patients who have good surveillance via monitoring by endoscopy *and* in patients adhering to a good diet.

While GI doctors put patients with Barrett's on a PPI, they rarely talk about dietary changes, possibly because they don't understand the role of pepsin in causing esophageal cancer, and are therefore not concerned about the negative impact of dietary acid. In *Dropping Acid: The Reflux Diet Cookbook & Cure,* I demonstrated that Barrett's esophagus biopsies show pepsin within the abnormal Barrett's tissue (see page 169 of that book). The purpose of an alkaline diet for Barrett's patients is to acid starve the pepsin-diseased areas.

I also believe that Barrett's is grossly over-diagnosed. For every three patients who come to me with the diagnosis, only one actually has it. This may have to do with the way the endoscopy and biopsies are performed. I perform TNE,[30] and because this examination is performed with the patient awake and swallowing normally, it is easy to see the anatomic landmarks that allow accurate biopsies to be obtained.

If you have been diagnosed with Barrett's, first get a second opinion and make sure the biopsies are done correctly. Given a choice of examination procedures, have a TNE rather than a sedated endoscopy. For more information see www.transnasalesophagoscopy.com. Second, remember that diet is vital, and PPIs are less so.[34]

The Barrett's patient should adhere to *Dr. Koufman's Acid Reflux Diet*, with the following modifications:

1. You should never drink another soft drink, including seltzer. Bottled and canned beverages are acid bombs for the esophagus and for your Barrett's.

2. You should always eat an early dinner. I recommend 6:00 p.m., assuming that you will go to bed after 11:00 p.m.

3. You should abstain from alcohol; it is one of the biggest reflux triggers.

4. Alkaline water should always be your beverage of choice. Make sure you have a steady supply available wherever you are.

5. You should avoid acidic foods like citrus except on rare occasions, and you should pH balance when you do consume acidic foods.

6. You should consider using Manuka honey lozenges, Manuka honey itself, or Manuka honey tea after meals, or at least after your evening meal. There is anecdotal evidence that Manuka honey is good for reflux and that it helps to heal the esophagus.

In summary, if you have Barrett's esophagus, get a second opinion, and focus on a healthy diet and lifestyle that keeps you reflux-free.

COOKING FOR LONGEVITY

CHAPTER 10

A Refluxer's Foodmap to Health

A s I said at the outset, this book is meant to be a companion to *Dropping Acid: The Reflux Diet Cookbook & Cure*. Its primary purpose is to continue to help refluxers after the fire has been put out, with the transition, maintenance, and longevity phases of *Dr. Koufman's Acid Reflux Diet*. This book is a continuation of the first book, and its recipes and suggestions will help you achieve lifelong relief from acid reflux symptoms, as well as weight loss and improved overall health.

Most of the recipes are vegan, and many are gluten-free and dairy-free at our patients' requests and because these constitute the cleanest and healthiest choices. All the recipes are pH balanced and nonacidic, and almost half are suitable for the detox phase of the reflux diet.

There is only a handful of meat recipes included. We assume that meat eaters will be able to prepare chicken, steak, or other meat without specific directions. Many of the recipes are Asian-inspired, as this is the forte of both Chef Philip and Sonia Huang. For some, this will mean purchasing new ingredients that you may never have used before. I had never cooked with sake, miso, or seaweed until I met Chef Philip. Incidentally, the type of Asian cooking presented in this book is already a proven longevity diet.

In the back of this book (page 228) there is a complete ingredient list, which is rarely provided in a cookbook. We have included this so that anyone with known reflux triggers can easily scan the list to avoid recipes that contain these foods.

We have listed the ingredients with the page numbers of the recipes that contain them to allow you to more easily find the foods/recipes that appeal to you. If you are a fish lover or adore the taste of cilantro, you can easily find recipes that use those ingredients.

We have also indicated "Possible Trigger" foods with the [PT] superscript. This designation means that the food is a reflux trigger for a significant proportion of my patients.

Questionably gluten-free items, those that "May or May Not Be Gluten-Free" depending on the brand, are indicated by the ^MMGF superscript, which means that you may need to closely read the package labels.

Finally, when you see a new-to-you item used in our recipes, we hope it will encourage you to take the plunge and try it, even if it is unfamiliar or has to be purchased online. As you will see, some "new" items, like kombu, are used in several recipes.

A reminder about pH balancing: In *Dropping Acid: The Reflux Diet Cookbook & Cure*, acidic foods and beverages are completely avoided. However, once a person has healed and the reflux is under control, even somewhat-acidic foods can be reintroduced. But please remember principles such as the following: If you are putting blueberries on your breakfast cereal, they are already pH balanced in the milk. But if you are eating the berries by themselves, or anything else that is moderately acidic, consider consuming something that is alkaline, too, like alkaline water. For more on this, see the section *pH Balancing* (page 59).

> Our recipes contain some acids and possible reflux trigger foods (PTs), including vinegar, wine, and berries. We believe that most people do NOT have these as trigger foods in the amounts used in the recipes. These ingredients are designated with a PT superscript. Finally, there are recipes in this book that are suitable for the detox diet, but most are not.

To Kombu or Not to Kombu? That Is the Question

The chances are that you have no idea what kombu is. I didn't. But perhaps kombu is somehow central to reflux-friendly, vegetarian cooking?

After Chef Philip and Sonia set to work, I was impressed with the great new recipes they were creating. One afternoon before leaving work, I was looking at the recipes and decided that I wanted to make the Miso Soup (page 109). The ingredients looked easily attainable until I saw 2 cups seaweed-mushroom stock. I turned a few pages, and there was the seaweed stock recipe (page 218): water, mushrooms, and kombu. KOMBU?

Well, I didn't have any kombu in my pantry, and after a telephone call to my neighborhood grocery store, I learned that they didn't have it either. Oh well. But wait! Kombu is ubiquitous in our recipes because it is in the basic vegetable stock (page 217) that is so often used in Chef Philip's reflux-friendly, vegan recipes. I was beside myself: To kombu or not to kombu? That was the question.

In working with a chef to provide as many reflux-friendly, vegetarian recipes as we could, choices had to be made. For example, I like chicken stock. In the past, I have used it a lot in my cooking, and thankfully, there are some organic store-bought brands that don't have sugar or chemicals in them. But, well, chicken stock is not vegetarian.

Vegetable stock is another matter, and Chef Philip had a challenge because store-bought vegetable stock almost always contains onion, which is a known reflux trigger for a lot of people. So, he had to create great flavor for a basic vegetable stock that is reflux-friendly as well.

Kombu is a kelp, a seaweed that is loaded with flavor and important in Asian cooking. I ordered it online, and clean, handpicked kombu was delivered to my door two days later.

As I have said, the hardest part of treating reflux is that everyone is different. This fact makes reflux-friendly, vegetarian, and gluten-free the default diet that pretty much everyone can live with. This book is full of really wonderful recipes, and I am impressed with Chef Philip's and Sonia's ability to combine flavors and textures in appealing new ways.

The recipes in this book provide a lot of options and ideas, especially when it comes to stocks and other cooking liquids, and it is not necessary to follow the recipes rigidly. For example, I have made Sonia's Steamed Sea Bass with Ginger & Soy (page 187) using chicken stock instead of wine and halibut instead of sea bass, and I poached it rather than steamed it.

Almost all of the seemingly unusual ingredients are available at specialty stores and online. So, I am suggesting that if you want to eat lean, clean, green, and alkaline, you should take a break from familiar ingredients and give them a try.

If I can kombu, so can you!

Food Definitions and Cooking Terms

Asafoetida. A traditional ingredient from India, produced from a tree resin. Used often in Indian, Hindu, and Jain cuisines that shun garlic and onion for religious reasons.

Chinkiang vinegar. A black rice vinegar from China, aged for several years, with a strong flavor.

Clove. This spice, commonly used in pumpkin pie, is the dried bud (unopened flower) of the clove tree.

Dairy-free (DF). DF means no animal milk products of any kind are consumed—not just cow (lactose), but also goat, sheep, etc. A dairy-free diet may or may not exclude eggs. (Vegans are dairy-free, but they also exclude all other animal products.)

Edamame are plain soybeans for cooking. Rarely found fresh in stores but easily found frozen.

Fermented black beans are used in many types of Chinese cooking and are easily found at Asian markets.

Garlic-infused olive oil. See *Kitchen Staples*, page 220. Garlic is a trigger for some refluxers, but it is the "meat" of the garlic that seems to cause the problem for most people. The infused oil is often not a trigger, thus providing the wonderful garlic flavor without the problem.

Gluten-free (GF). GF is generally accepted as less than 5–10 parts per million. We have tried our best to limit exposure to gluten by choosing mostly GF ingredients and recipes. Unfortunately, spices, even single-ingredient spices, may be contaminated. Therefore, with all spices, read the label, and specifically avoid those that contain "modified food starch." (Note: There are companies who advertise that their spices are GF but at the "less than 20 parts per million" level.)

> If you are GF for medical reasons, such as celiac disease, you (and not the authors) are responsible for checking all of your ingredients, including those recommended in this book.

Grapeseed oil. A flavorless oil derived from grapeseeds that can be used at very high temperatures, thus excellent for roasting and baking.

Hijiki. A seaweed used in Japan.

Julienne. A cutting technique, also called shoestring and matchstick, as it cuts a vegetable into the size of matchsticks. First cut 1/4-inch-thick slabs of your vegetable. Then lay the slabs on their side and cut 1/4-inch-wide slices.

Kanten. Agar derived from a seaweed. A traditional Japanese ingredient with uses similar to gelatin.

Kombu. A seaweed from Japan and Korea that is essential for flavoring many stocks and soups. Kombu is important in making vegetable stock for the recipes in this book because store-bought brands all contain onion.

Mirin. A sweet sake for cooking. Traditionally made from a slow rice-fermentation process, this was the established sweetener in Japan for centuries. There are two types of mirin on the market, hon-mirin (real mirin), which is aged, and aji-mirin, which is less flavorful and nutritious because it is not fermented. Obviously, we recommend hon-mirin, but substitute if you must.

Miso. A fermented soybean paste from Japan; various other types of fermented bean pastes are found throughout Asia. Miso comes in a wide variety of colors: the lighter misos are lower in salt and less aged, and the darker misos are stronger in flavor, saltier, and aged up to three years. Only use organic miso with no preservatives or alcohol added. For gluten-free diets, avoid mugi miso, which is made with barley, and for those who wish to avoid soy, use chickpea misos.

Mung dal. Dal are small, flavorful, and nutritious beans from India. Mung can be yellow or green and found whole or split.

Reflux detox diet. Strict, usually two-week, low-acid, low-fat diet; see page 47. Note: Most of the recipes in this book are for people whose reflux is not in the acute, decompensated stage—that is, many of the recipes are not for the reflux detox phase. See the Recipe Guide (page 223) for detox-friendly recipes (designated with a *). For foods that are acceptable during the detox phase, see page 48.

Sake. A traditional rice wine from Japan.

Shaoshing wine. A traditional aged rice wine from China. Dry sherry is a very good replacement. Sake is *not* a replacement! You must read the label, as some shaoshing is not gluten-free.

Sesame oil. Used for many types of Asian cooking. Use non-toasted sesame oil for stir-frying. This may be a trigger food for some people.

Shiitake. A mushroom originally from China, used widely in many styles of Asian cuisine. The dried ones are integral for making stocks.

Soy sauce. A traditional seasoning from various parts of Asia made from soybeans, salt, cultures, and, sometimes, wheat. For a gluten-free version, we suggest you use tamari.

Sumac. A lemony-flavored herb found in the Arab world. Good for refluxers, as lemon juice itself is usually a trigger, and sumac will impart a similar flavor.

Tahini. Sesame paste/butter from the Middle East.

Tamari. A Japanese soy sauce made with 100 percent soy; it is gluten-free.

Tempeh. A traditional cultured soy food from Indonesia that is high in protein and very flavorful and nutritious. One of Chef Philip's favorite ingredients!

Toasted sesame oil. Used to flavor dishes and added at the end of cooking. Never cook with toasted sesame oil, as it will burn immediately. Sesame oil is an uncommon, though possible, trigger food.

Vegan. Vegan diets exclude all animal products. Vegans also do not eat honey; if you are vegan, you may always substitute agave for honey.

Vegetable stock. We recommend that you make your own vegetable stock; see our recipe on page 217. Unfortunately, most store-bought vegetable stocks contain onions and sugar and are not gluten-free. Read the labels before purchasing.

Vegetarian. Unlike vegans (see above), some vegetarians eat eggs and dairy products such as milk and cheese.

Wakame. A seaweed used in many dishes in Japan and Korea.

BREAKFAST

Supa-Dupa Vegan Frittata

Vegan, Gluten-Free, Dairy-Free, Detox-Friendly
Makes 4 servings | 170 calories per serving

1 (16-ounce) package medium-firm tofu

½ cup soymilk

1¼ teaspoons sea salt

1 tablespoon cornstarch[MMGF]

½ teaspoon ground turmeric

1 teaspoon olive oil, plus as needed

2 cups mixed chopped vegetables (mushrooms, spinach, red pepper, or anything you like that is in season)

2 tablespoons chopped fresh basil

1 teaspoon fresh thyme, or ½ teaspoon dried thyme

1. Press the tofu by removing it from the package and placing it on a towel. Place another towel on the tofu and then a cutting board on top of this towel. Place a heavy can or another heavy item from your kitchen on the board. Let the tofu press for 10 minutes. Pressing the tofu will remove the water and allow it to absorb other flavors.
2. Place the tofu, soymilk, 1 teaspoon sea salt, cornstarch, and turmeric in a blender or food processor and purée until very smooth. Set aside.
3. Heat up a frying pan over medium heat and add the olive oil.
4. Add the vegetables and the remaining ¼ teaspoon sea salt.
5. Cook over medium heat, stirring regularly, until the vegetables are starting to wilt. Remove the cooked vegetables from the pan and set aside.
6. In the same frying pan, coat the surface with a little more olive oil.
7. Pour ¾ cup of the tofu-soymilk mixture into the pan, spreading evenly.
8. Cover and cook for 7 minutes, or until the surface is dry.
9. Add the cooked vegetables to the top of one side of the cooked tofu mixture.
10. Using a spatula, gently remove the frittata from the surface of the pan and fold one half over the side with the vegetables.
11. Sprinkle with the herbs and serve hot.

Notes: This frittata is very easy to make, and it is a simple yet flavorful breakfast food that I like to serve with the savory waffle (page 100) and a smoothie (pages 100–101). • This is the dish to make for brunch and for company, especially your vegetarian friends. –Chef Philip

Buckwheat Waffles

Vegan, Dairy-Free, Detox-Friendly
Makes 4 servings | 165 calories per serving

½ cup buckwheat flour

½ cup white flour^{NGF}

1 tablespoon palm sugar

¼ teaspoon baking soda^{MMGF}

½ teaspoon baking powder^{MMGF}

1 teaspoon vanilla extract

1 tablespoon grapeseed oil

1 cup soymilk (see note)

1. In one bowl, whisk together the dry ingredients.
2. In another bowl, whisk together the wet ingredients.
3. Add the wet ingredients to the dry and stir gently, leaving some lumps. (Overmixing will make the waffle rubbery.)
4. Pour ¾ cup of the batter into an oiled waffle iron and cook until done.

Notes: Only use soymilk made of two ingredients: organic soybeans and water. Any additives (sugars, gums, stabilizers) will simply destroy the healthy result you are seeking. • This is an outstanding breakfast dish with the wonderful flavor of buckwheat. • Serve with some fresh fruit and a bit of maple syrup for a nice, sweet breakfast, brunch, or even lunch. –Chef Philip

Gluten-Free Pumpkin Muffins

Vegetarian, Gluten-Free, Dairy-Free, Detox-Friendly
Makes 12 muffins | 130 calories per muffin

⅓ cup quinoa flour

½ cup quinoa flakes

1 teaspoon baking soda^{MMGF}

2 teaspoons baking powder^{MMGF}

1 teaspoon ground cinnamon

½ teaspoon ground ginger

¼ teaspoon ground cloves

2–3 tablespoons honey (optional)

2 eggs

2 ripe bananas, mashed

1 cup pumpkin purée (from can)

1. Preheat the oven to 400°F.
2. In one bowl, whisk together the quinoa flour, quinoa flakes, baking soda, baking powder, cinnamon, ginger, cloves, and salt.
3. In another bowl, whisk together the honey, eggs, bananas, and pumpkin.
4. Add the banana mixture to the flour mixture and stir gently.
5. Prepare a 12-muffin tin by spraying it with nonstick cooking spray (or coating it with grapeseed oil).
6. Divide the mixture between the muffin cups and bake for 25 minutes.

Notes: This recipe—a gluten-free muffin—was the number-one most-requested recipe. • The overall taste of this muffin is like pumpkin pie, and it will make your kitchen smell like Thanksgiving. • The honey does add sweetness, but the muffins are great without it—it's your choice whether to add the honey. • Be careful not to undercook or overcook. You can use the old toothpick method to see if the muffins are done: stick a toothpick into a muffin, and if it comes out "dry," without muffin mix on it, they are done. • We recommend a 12-muffin tin, because this makes relatively small muffins, and these muffins cook best when not too large. For this reason, a serving for breakfast may be two muffins. • If the muffin mixture only fills 10 or 11 of the muffin cups, that's fine, too. —Sonia

Gluten-Free Caramel Apple Muffins

Vegetarian, Gluten-Free
Makes 12 muffins | 125 calories per muffin

⅓ cup quinoa flour

½ cup quinoa flakes

1 teaspoon baking soda[MMGF]

2 teaspoons baking powder[MMGF]

1 teaspoon ground cinnamon

½ teaspoon ground nutmeg

½ teaspoon salt

½ cup caramel candy bits

1 teaspoon milk

1 cup diced red apple[PT]

2 tablespoons honey

2 eggs

2 very ripe bananas, mashed

1. Preheat the oven to 400°F.
2. In one bowl, whisk together the quinoa flour, quinoa flakes, baking soda, baking powder, cinnamon, nutmeg, and salt.
3. Heat a nonstick saucepan over medium heat and spray with nonstick cooking spray (or coat with grapeseed oil), then turn the heat to low. Add the caramel and milk and stir until the caramel is melted and smooth. Add the apples and stir for 1 minute. Remove from the heat and keep warm. (If the mixture hardens before use, you can microwave it in a microwave-safe bowl on high for 30 seconds.)
4. In another bowl, whisk together the honey, eggs, bananas, and caramel apple mixture.
5. Add the caramel mixture to the flour mixture and stir gently.
6. Prepare a 12-muffin tin by spraying it with nonstick cooking spray (or coating it with grapeseed oil).
7. Divide the mixture between the muffin cups and bake for 20–25 minutes.

Notes: This is for all of you with a sweet tooth. • This muffin is a sweet treat, so no more than two per person. • Great on-the-go breakfast with some fruit. • Because of the milk and caramel, this muffin is NOT dairy-free. • Incidentally, red apples are uncommonly a trigger food, so for most refluxers, these muffins are fine. • I cannot make these fast enough for my children. • As with the pumpkin muffins, if the mixture only fills 10 or 11 of the muffin cups, that's okay. —Sonia

Gluten-Free Morning Oatmeal

Vegan, Gluten-Free, Dairy-Free, Detox-Friendly
Makes 2 servings | 245 calories per serving

1 cup water

1 cup soymilk (almond or hemp milk work well, too)

Pinch of salt

1 cup gluten-free rolled oats^{MMGF}

2 tablespoons maple syrup

1. In a saucepan, heat up the water and soymilk with the salt.
2. Add the oats and bring to a boil, then lower the heat and cook for 10 minutes, stirring regularly.
3. Add the maple syrup before serving.

Notes: Fresh fruit—such as sliced bananas and berries—may be added after the oatmeal is cooked. • During the winter, you may want to use dried fruit, like raisins or apricots. • Chopped nuts, if not a trigger, can also be added. –Sonia

Corn Rye Savory Waffles

Vegan, Dairy-Free, Detox-Friendly
Makes 4–6 servings | 185 calories per serving

1 cup rye flour^{NGF}

1 cup cornmeal^{MMGF}

½ teaspoon sea salt

1 teaspoon baking powder^{MMGF}

½ teaspoon baking soda^{MMGF}

2 tablespoons grapeseed oil

2 cups soymilk (see note)

1. In one bowl, whisk together the dry ingredients.
2. In a separate bowl, whisk together the wet ingredients.
3. Add the wet ingredients to the dry and stir gently, leaving some lumps. (Over-mixing will make the waffle rubbery.)
4. Pour ¾ cup of the batter into an oiled waffle iron and cook until done.

Notes: Only use soymilk made of two ingredients: organic soybeans and water. Any additives (sugars, gums, stabilizers) will simply destroy the healthy result you are seeking. • This is a great brunch item, and it can be served with the Supa-Dupa Vegan Frittata (page 95). –Chef Philip

Berry Banana Smoothie

Vegan, Gluten-Free, Dairy-Free
Makes two 1-cup servings | 150 calories per serving

2 bananas

1 cup fresh or frozen berries^{PT}

½ cup water

½ cup crushed ice

1. Add all of the ingredients to a blender and blend until smooth.

Notes: Smoothies are flavorful, refreshing, filling, and an easy way to consume a fair amount of fruit. • Smoothies are great for breakfast or as a snack. • As an option, you may add a pinch of cinnamon or allspice. –Chef Philip

A Very Peachy Smoothie

Vegan, Gluten-Free, Dairy-Free
Makes two 1-cup servings | 190 calories per serving

2 bananas

2 ripe peaches,[PT] peeled, halved, and pitted

½ cup water

½ cup crushed ice

1. Add all of the ingredients to a blender and blend until smooth.

Notes: As an option you can add ¼ teaspoon cinnamon or replace the peaches with pears or apples or a combination. —Chef Philip

Pear & Melon Smoothie

Vegan, Gluten-Free, Dairy-Free, Detox-Friendly
Makes two 1-cup servings | 140 calories per serving

1 banana

1 pear, peeled and cored

1 cup cubed fresh cantaloupe or honeydew melon

½ cup crushed ice

1. Add all of the ingredients to a blender and blend until smooth.

Notes: For smoothness and for reflux relief, consider adding a 2-inch piece (the inside part) of peeled aloe vera. • Actually, this option is good for all smoothies! • Do not use bottled or prepared aloe vera, just the fresh leaf. —Chef Philip

Basil Omelet

Vegetarian, Gluten-Free, Dairy-Free
Makes 2 servings | 215 calories per serving

6 egg whites

3 egg yolks

½ cup whole basil leaves, without stems

½ teaspoon salt or to taste

2 tablespoons olive oil

1 teaspoon toasted sesame oil[PT]

(optional)

1. Beat the egg whites and yolks with the basil leaves, then add salt to taste.
2. Heat both oils together in a small pan over medium-high heat. Add the egg mixture and cook undisturbed until the bottom is lightly browned, then carefully flip to cook the other side until done.

Notes: The best foods are often the simple ones. • An interesting fact: This omelet is often served to new moms in China to help them recover from childbirth. –Sonia

Everyday Lox Omelet

Gluten-Free, Dairy-Free
Makes 1 serving | 185 calories per serving

2 slices Nova Scotia smoked salmon (lox)

3 eggs

1. Cut the smoked salmon into small pieces.
2. Crack the eggs into a small bowl, discarding two of the yolks, and lightly whisk with a fork.
3. Heat up a frying pan over medium heat.
4. Spray with nonstick cooking spray (or coat with grapeseed oil) and add the eggs.
5. Cook the eggs undisturbed until almost done, then flip with a spatula.
6. Place the lox on the omelet, then fold.
7. Cook 1 more minute and serve.

Notes: This is a staple breakfast item that is easy to cook yourself or to order out. When I get to work, I often get this omelet from the bodega in my building • It doesn't get much simpler than, "I'll have a three-egg omelet with one yolk and lox." –Dr. Jamie

Egg White Wrap with Dill or Basil

Vegetarian, Dairy-Free, Detox-Friendly
Makes 2 servings | 270 calories per serving

6 egg whites

2 tablespoons chopped fresh dill or basil

¼ teaspoon salt

1 tablespoon olive oil

2 flour tortillas^{NGF}

1. Beat the egg whites with the dill or basil and the salt.
2. Heat the oil in a small pan over medium-high heat. Add the egg mixture and scramble until cooked through.
3. Heat each tortilla in a skillet for 30 seconds to soften and to bring out the flavor.
4. Divide the egg mixture between the tortillas and roll.

Notes: Use dill or basil, not both. • If you like, you could also add smoked salmon (lox) with the dill (for a non-vegetarian option) or tomatoes with the basil. —Sonia

Rice Porridge with Chicken

Gluten-Free, Dairy-Free, Detox-Friendly
Makes 4 servings | 325 calories per serving

4 dried shiitake mushrooms

2 tablespoons olive oil

1 teaspoon minced fresh ginger

½ pound ground chicken

4 cups chicken stock (page 217)

2 cups cooked white rice

Salt to taste

2 tablespoons chopped fresh cilantro

1 teaspoon sesame oil[PT] (optional; see note)

1. In warm water soak the mushrooms until soft.
2. Rinse the mushrooms and pat dry.
3. Remove the stems and thinly slice the caps.
4. Heat the olive oil in a pan over medium-high heat. Add the ginger and sauté for 1 minute. Add the mushrooms and ground chicken and sauté until the chicken is browned. Remove from the heat and set aside.
5. Bring the chicken stock to a boil in a saucepan over medium-high heat.
6. Add the cooked white rice and return to a boil, then reduce the heat to low and cook until soft, about 15 minutes.
7. Add the chicken and mushroom mixture and cook another 5 minutes, then add salt to taste.
8. Pour into bowls, top with the cilantro, drizzle with the sesame oil, and serve.

Notes: If the sesame oil is omitted, this dish is detox-friendly. • This is a common Taiwanese breakfast dish. • The chicken may be substituted with leftover vegetables, another meat, or any fish, and even the rice may be leftovers. • Every grandma in China and Japan will have her own version of this dish, and probably never measure anything. • Once you start, this may also become one of your go-to recipes. • Have fun experimenting! –Sonia

SOUPS

Miso Soup

Vegan, Gluten-Free, Dairy-Free, Detox-Friendly
Makes 2 servings | 50 calories per serving

2 cups seaweed-mushroom stock (page 218)
¼ cup combination of chopped vegetables, tofu, mushrooms, and rehydrated
  wakame seaweed
4 teaspoons miso

1. Bring the stock to a simmer in a saucepan.
2. Add the vegetables, tofu, mushrooms, and seaweed and cook for 1 minute.
3. Remove from the heat.
4. Remove 2 tablespoons stock and add to a bowl with the miso. Whisk
   together to dissolve the miso.
5. Add the miso and stock mixture back to the rest of the soup.
6. Stir and serve immediately.

Notes: Miso soup is one of the world's healthiest foods. • Many active, healthy octogenarians in Japan have been eating miso soup with every meal, breakfast included, all of their lives! • Use your favorite seasonal fresh vegetables. • This soup is simple and fast to make with very flavorful results. • Make your stock in advance and keep it in the fridge or freezer, and then you can make miso soup in the amount of time it takes to boil water; it is that simple to do. • There are different types of miso, from very light to very dark. The darker the miso, the more aged and saltier it is, and thus, the more intense tasting. • The lighter ones are sweeter. • Lighter miso is generally used in warmer weather and darker miso in colder weather. • Use any miso that is naturally aged and has no added preservatives or alcohol. —Chef Philip

Egg Drop Soup

Gluten-Free, Dairy-Free, Detox-Friendly
Makes 4 servings | 130 calories per serving

4 cups chicken stock (page 217)

¼ teaspoon salt

¼ teaspoon minced fresh ginger
(not bottled)

3 tablespoons water

1½ tablespoons cornstarch[MMGF]

4 egg whites

Chopped fresh cilantro, for garnish
(optional)

1. Heat the chicken stock in a saucepan over medium-high heat.
2. Add the salt and ginger and bring to a boil.
3. In a small bowl, stir the water and cornstarch together until smooth and set aside.
4. Whisk the egg whites in a small bowl, then set aside.
5. Drizzle the egg a little at a time into the boiling broth while stirring the broth.
6. Gradually stir in the cornstarch mixture until the desired consistency is reached.
7. Serve hot topped with cilantro.

Notes: In Taiwan, traditionally a family meal consists of three main dishes and a soup, or five main dishes and a soup. • This would be a great start for any family meal. • This classic and traditional Chinese dish can be made vegetarian by using vegetable stock in place of chicken stock. • The addition of cilantro brightens up this dish a lot. —Sonia

Tuscan White Bean Soup

Vegan, Gluten-Free, Dairy-Free
Makes 4 servings | 400 calories per serving

¼ cup olive oil

1 stalk celery, diced

1 carrot, diced

1 cup fresh shelled peas

2 teaspoons sea salt

2 bay leaves

1 teaspoon dried oregano

1 teaspoon dried thyme

½ teaspoon dried rosemary

¼ cup dry white wine[PT]

4 cups seaweed-mushroom or vegetable stock (pages 217–218)

1 can white beans, rinsed and drained

1 cup chopped fresh basil

¼ cup chopped fresh parsley (preferably Italian)

1. In a large soup pot, add the olive oil.
2. Add the vegetables, salt, bay leaves, and dried herbs and cook for 10 minutes.
3. Add the white wine and cook for another 5 minutes.
4. Add the stock and beans, bring to a simmer, then season to taste.
5. Remove the bay leaves and add the basil and parsley.

Notes: This is a classic Northern Italian soup. • Make this a one-pot meal: add 1–2 cups cooked pasta (bowtie or orzo is excellent) to the finished soup. • For lunch, try this soup with a salad and a hearty bread (if you are a gluten eater). —Chef Philip

Shrimp & Tofu Soup

Gluten-Free, Dairy-Free
Makes 4–6 servings | 270 calories per serving

2 tablespoons olive oil

4 (⅛-inch-thick) slices fresh ginger
  (no need to peel)

½ pound uncooked shrimp, peeled,
  deveined, and coarsely chopped
  (¼- to ½-inch pieces)

½ teaspoon rice wine[PT]

6 cups chicken stock (page 217)

½ cup sliced canned bamboo shoots

1 (12-ounce) package soft tofu, cut into
  1-inch cubes

2 ounces prosciutto,[PT] diced

¼ cup water

¼ cup cornstarch[MMGF]

3 egg whites, beaten

Salt to taste

1 tablespoon sesame oil[PT]

2 tablespoons chopped fresh cilantro

1. Heat the olive oil in a pan over medium-high heat. Sauté the ginger for 2 minutes.
2. Add the shrimp and rice wine and cook until opaque. Remove from the heat, discard the ginger, and set the shrimp aside.
3. Bring the chicken stock to a boil in a saucepan over medium-high heat. Add the bamboo shoot, tofu, prosciutto, and shrimp and bring back to a boil.
4. Whisk together the water and cornstarch and slowly add the mixture to the pot while stirring constantly.
5. Slowly drizzle in the egg whites while stirring. Add salt to taste.
6. Drizzle with the sesame oil, top with the cilantro, and serve.

Notes: This is an old family recipe passed down from my grandmother. • The fresh shrimp and soft tofu provide a pleasingly contrasting texture. • A light and flavorful soup that is very easy to make. • Get the prosciutto cut for you at the deli counter of your market; two ¼-inch-thick pieces should be close to 2 ounces. Before you dice the prosciutto, remove the fat first. • The amounts of sesame oil and wine are small enough that they are not likely to trigger reflux. • Note that cornstarch may or may not be gluten-free; check the brand and packaging label. –Sonia

Wonderful Wild Mushroom Soup

Vegan, Gluten-Free, Dairy-Free
Makes 4 servings | 225 calories per serving

⅓ cup raw pine nuts

4 cups vegetable stock (page 217)

3 tablespoons olive oil

1 stalk celery, diced

1 pound wild mushrooms, chopped
(see note)

1 sprig fresh thyme

10 fresh sage leaves, chopped

2 teaspoons sea salt

2 tablespoons dry sherry^{PT}

Chopped fresh parsley, for garnish

1. Blend the pine nuts and stock in a blender until puréed and totally smooth. Set aside.
2. In a hot soup pot, add the olive oil.
3. Add the celery and mushrooms, thyme, sage, and sea salt, and cook until the mushrooms start to wilt.
4. Add the sherry and cook until the alcohol flavor is gone.
5. Pour in the blended pine nut and stock mixture and bring to a simmer, stirring often.
6. Season to taste and garnish with fresh parsley.

Notes: Use whatever mushrooms are in season and available or that you prefer.
• Wild mushrooms are more flavorful than cultivated ones, but if wild mushrooms are unavailable, you can use regular store-bought shiitake, cremini, or portobello mushrooms, or a combination; indeed, a combination may be better than just one type. • Clean mushrooms carefully to get rid of all grit. • I prefer to make this soup with chanterelle mushrooms, which I forage in the Oakland hills. –Chef Philip

Caribbean Pumpkin Soup

Vegan, Gluten-Free, Dairy-Free
Makes 4 servings | 300 calories per serving

There are two steps to this recipe, the stock and the soup; the stock can be made in advance.

Stock

1 small sugar pie pumpkin (also called pie pumpkin)

1 stalk celery, coarsely chopped

1 carrot, peeled and coarsely chopped

1 large onion,^PT peeled and coarsely chopped

1 medium-size potato, peeled and coarsely chopped

2 whole cloves

1 stick cinnamon

1 sprig fresh thyme

5 allspice berries

2 quarts water

1 teaspoon sea salt

Directions for the Stock

1. Peel the pumpkin and remove the seeds and reserve; save the meat of the pumpkin for the soup; see pages 114–115.
2. Place the pumpkin peel and seeds in a stockpot, along with the celery, carrot, onion, potato, cloves, cinnamon, thyme, allspice, water, and salt.
3. Bring to a boil, then reduce the heat, cover, and let simmer for 2 hours. The liquid will reduce by half.
4. Strain the stock and reserve; discard the solid parts.

Soup

2 tablespoons olive oil

Pumpkin meat reserved from making stock, diced

1 small parsnip, diced

1 carrot, diced

1 small potato, diced

1 stalk celery, diced

1 teaspoon sea salt

2 tablespoons chopped fresh parsley

Directions for the Soup

1. In a hot soup pot, add the olive oil, then add the vegetables and sea salt.
2. Over medium heat, stirring often, cook the vegetables for 10 minutes, adding a little stock if they start to stick.
3. Purée half the vegetables with the stock in a blender, leaving the remaining vegetables intact.
4. Add the puréed vegetables and stock to the solid vegetables and bring to a boil over medium heat, stirring regularly.
5. Garnish with the chopped parsley.

Notes: Optional: add one habanero pepper,[PT] left whole, to the stock (if not a trigger food and if you're not on the detox diet). • There is a wide variety of pumpkins on the market. Use small orange pumpkins (about 8-inch diameter) for this soup, known as pie pumpkins or sugar pumpkins. • Butternut squash can be used as an alternative to pumpkin. • Pumpkin is a wonderful vegetable with incredibly diverse uses, both savory and sweet. • Native to the American continents, pumpkin was widely used by native cultures for its incredible flavor and nutrition as well as for decorative uses. • I learned this recipe from friends from Jamaica while a graduate student in Florida. • This soup also makes use of one of Jamaica's indigenous ingredients, allspice. • This dish contains onion, which is a reflux trigger for many people. –Chef Philip

Asparagus Miso Chowder

Vegan, Gluten-Free, Dairy-Free, Detox-Friendly
Makes 4 servings | 230 calories per serving

3 medium-size red potatoes or other creamy potato, diced into ½-inch cubes

2 tablespoons olive oil 1 pound asparagus, trimmed and cut into ½-inch pieces

¼ cup white miso (preferably Saikyo miso; see Food Definitions, page 90)

4 cups vegetable or seaweed-mushroom stock (page 217–218

½ teaspoon smoked paprika,[PT] for garnish (optional)

1. In a soup pot, sauté the potatoes in the olive oil over medium heat until the potatoes are soft.
2. Add the asparagus and cook for 3 more minutes.
3. Place half of the cooked vegetables in a blender and add the miso and stock.
4. Purée until very smooth.
5. Place the purée back into the pot with the solid cooked vegetables and stir to combine.
6. Serve in bowls and garnish each with a small amount of smoked paprika.

Notes: Omit the paprika and this dish is detox-friendly. • Saikyo is the sweetest white miso; if unavailable, any other light miso can substitute. • Asparagus is a wonderful fresh vegetable with a short growing season. • During the three months it is available, I use this chowder in a wide variety of contexts, and I have even developed desserts using it. • This is an easy-to-make spring soup. • If the paprika is omitted, this dish is suitable for the detox diet. —Chef Philip

Basic Indian Bean Soup

Vegan, Gluten-Free, Dairy-Free, Detox-Friendly
Makes 4 servings | 210 calories per serving

6 cups water

2 tablespoons olive oil

⅔ cup dried whole mung beans

1 tablespoon minced fresh ginger

½ teaspoon ground turmeric (see note)

2 teaspoons ground coriander

1 teaspoon cumin seeds

1 teaspoon brown mustard seeds^{MMGF}

1 ½ teaspoons salt

¼ teaspoon asafoetida^{MMGF}

3 tablespoons chopped fresh cilantro

1. In a soup pot, bring the water to a boil.
2. Add ½ tablespoon olive oil and the mung beans, ginger, turmeric, and coriander.
3. Bring to a simmer, cover, lower the heat, and cook for 1 hour and 15 minutes.
4. In a hot frying pan or wok, add the remaining 1 ½ tablespoons olive oil.
5. Add the cumin seeds and mustard seeds and stir-fry for 30 seconds.
6. Add this to the dal soup, then add the salt, asafoetida, and cilantro.
7. Whisk the soup together to combine.
8. Cover for 1 minute and then serve hot.

Notes: If you can get fresh turmeric, by all means use it! Replace the ground turmeric with 1 tablespoon grated fresh turmeric. Wash your hands, knife, and utensils immediately after using fresh turmeric, as it will stain everything. • I love this soup! This is an every-week dish in my home. • So simple to make with such delightful results in texture and flavor. • You can use a variety of lentils (green, red, and yellow) along with the mung beans for some different tastes and textures. • Years ago, I asked some friends from India for the best way to learn about Indian food, and they said to start with dal. Here is the first one I learned. —Chef Philip

Southern Black-Eyed Pea Soup

Vegan, Gluten-Free, Dairy-Free
Makes 4 servings | 155 calories per serving

1 cup black-eyed peas, soaked overnight
  or for at least 8 hours
1 tablespoon olive oil
1 carrot, diced
1 stalk celery, diced
1 bunch collard greens, chopped
1 teaspoon dried thyme

1 teaspoon dried oregano
4 cups seaweed-mushroom or vegetable
stock (page 218)
½ teaspoon sea salt
2 tablespoons balsamic vinegar [PT, MMGF]
¼ cup chopped fresh parsley

1. Drain and rinse the soaked black-eyed peas.
2. In a hot soup pot, add the olive oil.
3. Add the carrot, celery, and collards and sauté for 5 minutes.
4. Add the thyme, oregano, black-eyed peas, and stock and bring to a boil.
5. Lower the heat, cover, and simmer for 25 minutes, or until the black-eyed peas are soft.
6. Stir in the salt, vinegar, and parsley.

Notes: While working on graduate studies at the Florida State University School of Music, I began organic gardening and learned more about Southern vegetables. • Black-eyed peas became a favorite, and I started to learn a wide variety of dishes to prepare using this flavorful and highly nutritious bean. • Black-eyed peas are native to West Africa; they were brought to the southeast United States by slaves and have become a staple of Southern cuisine. • Like all bean soups, this soup tastes even better the second day, as all the flavors have merged. This soup has a relatively long shelf life. –Chef Philip

Chicken-Stuffed Cucumber Soup

Gluten-Free, Dairy-Free
Makes 8 servings | 230 calories per serving

Marinade

1 egg white

1 tablespoon minced fresh ginger

2 tablespoons water

1 teaspoon salt

1 teaspoon tamari (gluten-free soy sauce)

¼ teaspoon honey

1 tablespoon cornstarch^{MMGF}

Dash of toasted sesame oil^{PT} (see note)

Soup

1 pound ground chicken

2 tablespoons cornstarch^{MMGF}

2 medium cucumbers, peeled, seeded to make a hollow area, and sliced cross wise into 2-inch pieces

8 cups chicken stock (page 217)

2 (¼-inch-thick) slices peeled fresh ginger, diced

1 teaspoon salt

8 shiitake or portobello mushrooms, trimmed and sliced

10 sprigs fresh cilantro, chopped, for garnish

4 teaspoons sesame oil^{PT}

1. Combine all of the marinade ingredients in a bowl.
2. Add the ground chicken, mix well, and let marinate for 5 minutes.
3. Lightly dust the cornstarch inside the cucumber pieces.
4. Stuff each hollowed-out area of cucumber with chicken mixture.
5. Bring the chicken stock to a boil in a soup pot over medium-high heat, then add the sliced ginger and salt.
6. Add the stuffed cucumber pieces, bring back to a boil, then lower the heat to medium-low and gently boil for 10–15 minutes, or until the chicken is cooked through.
7. Add the mushrooms and simmer for 1 minute.
8. Serve hot with the chopped cilantro and a drizzle of sesame oil.

Notes: Substitute extra-virgin olive oil if sesame oil is a trigger. • This may take a little bit of effort to make, but it is worth it. • The beautifully presented little gems of sweet cucumber stuffed with savory meat are just delightful. • Makes an impressive dish to serve at a party. –Sonia

Roasted Cauliflower &
Watercress Miso Chowder

Vegan, Gluten-Free, Dairy-Free
Makes 4 servings | 300 calories per serving

½ pound (any) potatoes (usually 2 medium), peeled, ½-inch dice

1 stalk celery, diced

1 carrot, minced

1 head cauliflower, diced

½ teaspoon sea salt

1 tablespoon safflower oil

3 cups vegetable stock (page 217)

⅓ cup raw pistachios[PT]

¼ cup white miso (optional; see Food Definitions, page 90)

1 small bunch watercress

4 teaspoons high-quality olive oil, for garnish

1. Preheat the oven to 425°F.
2. In a roasting pan, add the potatoes, celery, carrots, and cauliflower. Sprinkle with the sea salt and safflower oil. Cover with foil and roast for 30 minutes.
3. Add half the roasted vegetables to a blender.
4. Add the stock, pistachios, miso, and watercress to the blender and purée until very smooth.
5. Add the purée to a pot, along with the solid cooked vegetables.
6. Bring to a simmer but do not boil!
7. Serve in bowls and garnish each with up to a teaspoon of very good olive oil.

Notes: As a child growing up in Brooklyn, I loved the fresh cauliflower that was found in upstate New York during the summer. This infatuation has only grown over the years as I learn more and more dishes to create with this versatile vegetable. • This soup is very popular on my catering menus and has been a huge hit at my underground restaurant in Oakland. • Basil can be substituted for watercress. • This soup is great for a winter evening because it is thick and hearty. • When you prepare the cauliflower and potatoes, remember that these need to be bite-size. • By the way, this chowder is probably detox-friendly, because of all of the different kinds of nuts, pistachios are the least common reflux trigger. —Chef Philip

Middle Eastern Garbanzo Tahini Soup

Vegan, Gluten-Free, Dairy-Free
Makes 4 servings | 280 calories per serving

½ cup garbanzo beans, soaked overnight or for at least 8 hours

4 cups water

10 cloves garlic^{PT}

1 bay leaf

¼ cup tahiniPT

2 tablespoons balsamic vinegar ^{PT, MMGF}

2 tablespoons olive oil

2 carrots, sliced on the diagonal

1½ teaspoons sea salt

2 teaspoons dried oregano

1 pound fresh spinach, washed and chopped

5 cups vegetable or seaweed-mushroom stock (pages 217–218)

2 teaspoons sumac^{PT}

¼ cup chopped fresh parsley

1 tablespoon lemon zest

1. Drain and rinse the soaked garbanzos and place in a soup pot.
2. Cover with the water, then add the garlic cloves and bay leaf. Bring to a boil, lower the heat, cover, and simmer for 45 minutes, or until the garbanzos are tender.
3. Drain the garbanzos, removing the bay leaf and garlic. Set the garbanzos aside.
4. In a separate bowl, mix the tahini with the balsamic vinegar to make a paste, adding cold water as needed. Set aside.
5. In a hot soup pot, add the olive oil.
6. Add the carrot, salt, oregano, and spinach and cook for 8 minutes.
7. Add the stock and bring to a simmer.
8. Add the tahini-vinegar paste and blend well, then add the garbanzos.
9. Bring back to a simmer and add the sumac and parsley.
10. Taste!! Add salt or the lemon zest.

Notes: This dish only works if garlic is not a trigger food for you. • The Arabic world has provided so many wonderful ingredients, such as the sumac, garbanzos, and tahini used in this recipe. • These ingredients traveled the Silk Road and beyond centuries ago and have been incorporated into various other cuisines as a result. • This dish contains ingredients that may be reflux triggers for some people. —Chef Philip

Pork & Lily Bud Soup

Gluten-Free, Dairy-Free
Makes 4 servings | 350 calories per serving

2 ounces dried lily buds

5 cups chicken stock (page 217)

1 pound white pork, cut into 1-inch cubes

1 tablespoon rice wine[PT]

Salt to taste

1. Rinse the lily buds and tie each into a knot, then soak in warm water until soft, 15–30 minutes.
2. Heat the chicken stock in a soup pot over medium-high heat until boiling.
3. Add the pork, lily buds, and rice wine and bring back to a boil. Reduce the heat to a simmer and cover the pot.
4. Cook until the pork is tender, about 35–40 minutes.
5. Season with salt to taste.

Notes: Dried lily buds were once considered a luxury, served usually during the summer to lower one's internal heat, also called one's "chi." They are also thought to be good for people with breathing problems. • Both the flower and the bulb are edible. • Today, lily buds are inexpensive and easy to find. If they are not in your grocery store, you can find them online. –Sonia

Chinese Tofu Watercress Soup

Vegan, Gluten-Free, Dairy-Free
Makes 4 servings | 145 calories per serving

2 tablespoons safflower oil

2 (1 by ⅛-inch) slices fresh ginger

1 tablespoon palm sugar

¼ cup tamari (gluten-free soy sauce)

1–2 cups chopped watercress

4 cups seaweed-mushroom stock
  (page 218

8 ounces medium-firm tofu, cut into
  ½-inch cubes

1 tablespoon chinkiang vinegar[PT, MMGF]
  or rice vinegar [PT, MMGF]

1. In a hot wok, add the oil.
2. Add the ginger and stir-fry for 30 seconds.
3. Add the palm sugar and tamari and stir-fry for another 30 seconds.
4. Add the watercress, stock, and tofu and bring to a simmer.
5. Add the vinegar.
6. Season to taste: add tamari if salt is needed, and add vinegar if more tartness is needed.
7. Remove the ginger slices before serving.

Notes: This Chinese soup is very easy and fast to create with satisfying results, perfect for an evening when you want a hot soup and have very little time to produce it. • For variations, replace the watercress with 1–2 cups (chopped) of any of the following greens for a similar yet unique soup: spinach, choy sum, basil, collards, cilantro. –Chef Philip

Corn Chowder

Vegan, Gluten-Free, Dairy-Free, Detox-Friendly
Makes 4 servings | 195 calories per serving

2 tablespoons olive oil

2 teaspoons sea salt

Kernels from 2 ears corn

2 medium potatoes, ¼-inch dice

1 large carrot, ¼-inch dice

1 stalk celery, finely diced

1 cup fresh shelled peas

4 cups seaweed-mushroom stock
(page 218)

1 sprig fresh rosemary

2 tablespoons chopped fresh parsley

¼ cup chopped fresh basil

Smoked paprika,[PT] for garnish (optional;
see note)

1. In a hot soup pot, add the olive oil, sea salt, and all the vegetables. Sauté over medium heat for 10 minutes.
2. Add the stock and rosemary sprig and bring to a boil, then reduce the heat and let simmer for 3 minutes, or until the vegetables are fully cooked.
3. Add the parsley and basil and adjust the salt if needed.
4. Garnish with smoked paprika.

Note: If the paprika is omitted, this dish is detox-friendly. • This soup is best in the late summer and fall when fresh corn is at its best. • It's hard to imagine anyone not loving this hearty, vegan, creamy soup, laden with different-colored and different-textured vegetables. • Add a green salad and some hearty bread for a delightful fall lunch. —Chef Philip

Borscht

Vegan, Gluten-Free, Dairy-Free

Makes 4 servings | 75 calories per serving

2 pounds purple beets (3 large), peeled, ½-inch dice

1 tablespoon grapeseed oil

1 teaspoon sea salt

2 tablespoons chopped fresh dill

3 cups water

1-inch piece fresh horseradish,^{PT} grated, or 1 teaspoon dried horseradish powder^{PT}

2 teaspoons balsamic vinegar ^{PT, MMGF} (optional)

1. Preheat the oven to 425°F.
2. Place the beets in a roasting pan with the oil and salt. Stir to coat well. Cover and roast for 30 minutes.
3. Combine the roasted beets, dill, water, horseradish, and balsamic vinegar in a blender and purée until smooth.
4. Chill and serve very cold in the summer, or bring to a simmer and serve hot in the winter.

Notes: Classic Eastern European soup with many variations found throughout areas inhabited by Ashkenazi Jews. • Ice-cold borscht is incredibly refreshing in the summer, whereas hot borscht is warm and filling in the winter. • In the winter, add some sautéed cabbage to the finished soup, or for tartness, add sauerkraut (page 221). –Chef Philip

SALADS

Hummus Salad

Vegan, Gluten-Free, Dairy-Free
Makes 4 servings | 290 calories per serving

1 (16-ounce) can garbanzo beans, drained and rinsed

2 tablespoons high-quality olive oil or garlic-infused olive oil^PT (preferable; page 220)

2 tablespoons lemon zest

3 tablespoons tahini^PT

1 teaspoon ground cumin

½ teaspoon ground coriander

1 teaspoon sea salt

1 teaspoon sumac^PT

2 tablespoons chopped fresh dill, or 1 teaspoon dried dill

1 cucumber, thinly sliced

1 carrot, grated

½ cup alfalfa or radish sprouts

1. In a food processor, add the beans, olive oil, lemon zest, tahini, cumin, coriander, salt, sumac, and dill and purée until very smooth.
2. Transfer the hummus to a bowl. Place the sliced cucumbers around the sides, pile the grated carrots in the middle, and top with the sprouts.

Notes: Use garlic-infused olive oil instead of plain olive oil, if garlic is not a trigger food, for best flavor. More flavor can be added via sweet paprika or smoked paprika, if desired. • Hummus is found throughout the Arabic, Middle Eastern, and Mediterranean world, with a wide variety of recipes from region to region and from home to home. • Hummus is one of the many flavorful traditional dishes from around the world that is vegan by coincidence. –Chef Philip

Spanish Bean Salad

Vegan, Gluten-Free, Dairy-Free
Makes 6 servings | 290 calories per serving

¼ pound green beans, trimmed and cut into ½-inch pieces

1 (16-ounce) can garbanzo beans

1 (16-ounce) can kidney beans

1 (16-ounce) can black-eyed peas

1 large carrot, grated

1 teaspoon dried rosemary

2 teaspoons dried oregano

1 teaspoon dried thyme

3 tablespoons olive oil

3 tablespoons sherry vinegar [PT, MMGF]

2 teaspoons sea salt

1 teaspoon mustard powder

1 tablespoon lemon zest

¼ cup chopped fresh parsley

1. Blanch the green beans by dropping them in boiling water for 5 seconds. Rinse under cold water and drain.
2. Rinse the 3 cans of beans well and drain.
3. Place all of the ingredients in a large bowl and mix well.
4. Let marinate for 2 hours before serving.

Notes: The combination of the dried herbs, olive oil, and sherry vinegar create a very refreshing salad for all seasons. • Like all bean salads and soups, make this a day ahead to allow the flavors to fully develop and blend. —Chef Philip

French Lentil Salad

Vegan, Gluten-Free, Dairy-Free
Makes 4 servings | 165 calories per serving

1 cup green lentils, soaked overnight or for at least 8 hours

1 quart boiling water

1 tablespoon olive oil

1 carrot, diced

1 stalk celery, diced

1 cup fresh shelled peas

½ teaspoon dried thyme

½ teaspoon dried oregano

½ teaspoon dried marjoram

½ teaspoon dried rosemary

1 teaspoon sea salt

2 tablespoons lemon zest

¼ cup chopped fresh parsley or basil

2 tablespoons balsamic vinegar [PT, MMGF]

1. Drain and rinse the soaked lentils.
2. Cook the lentils in the boiling water for 10 minutes, or until the lentils are soft. Do not overcook!
3. Drain the lentils well and set aside in a bowl.
4. In a hot frying pan, add the olive oil, vegetables, dried herbs, and salt. Sauté for 5 minutes, or until the vegetables are cooked.
5. Add the cooked vegetables to the cooked lentils, then add the lemon zest, parsley, and balsamic vinegar and toss well to combine.

Notes: Lentils are an inexpensive, versatile source of vegetable protein that can be used in an infinite number of ways. —Chef Philip

Hijiki Seaweed Salad

Vegan, Gluten-Free, Dairy-Free
Makes 4 servings | 85 calories per serving

½ ounce dried hijiki

1 quart water

1 carrot, julienned

2 tablespoons sake[PT]

2 tablespoons mirin[PT]

2 tablespoons tamari (gluten-free soy
sauce)

1 cup seaweed-mushroom stock
(page 218)

½ cup fresh or frozen shelled edamame

1 tablespoon toasted sesame seeds[PT]
(optional)

1. Reconstitute the hijiki by soaking it in the water for 30 minutes. Drain and rinse.
2. Place the hijiki with the carrot, sake, mirin, tamari, and stock in a pot and bring to a simmer.
3. Cover, lower the heat, and cook for 30 minutes.
4. Add the edamame and cook another 10 minutes, adding more stock if needed.
5. Garnish with the toasted sesame seeds.

Notes: Hijiki is a very inexpensive seaweed found in the oceans off the coast of Japan. It is good to consume a small amount of sea vegetables daily for their nutritional value. • This is a very easy side dish using this nutritious sea vegetable. Hijiki has a strong, intense flavor, so usually small servings of this dish are offered. — Chef Philip

Cucumber Wakame Salad

Vegan, Gluten-Free, Dairy-Free
Makes 4 servings | 20 calories per serving

1 cucumber, cut into ⅛-inch-thick slices

½ teaspoon salt

2 tablespoons dried wakame

1 cup cold water

1 carrot, grated

2 teaspoons rice vinegar [PT, MMGF]

1 teaspoon mirin[PT]

1 teaspoon tamari (gluten-free soy sauce)

1. Place the cucumber slices in a colander set over a bowl, sprinkle with the salt, and massage it into the slices. Let the cucumber sit in the colander for 30 minutes, then rinse and drain.
2. Meanwhile, rehydrate the wakame by placing it in the cold water for 15 minutes. Drain and squeeze excess water out of the wakame.
3. Place the cucumber and wakame with the remaining ingredients in a bowl and gently mix. Serve immediately.

Notes: Another very simple side dish from Japan involving sea and land vegetables. • Wakame is one of the most popular sea vegetables, and it shows up on many daily menus in Japan and Korea. • Wakame is harvested in the Pacific and, like other seaweeds, is highly nutritious and very inexpensive. —Chef Philip

Roasted Portobello Mushroom Salad

Vegan, Gluten-Free, Dairy-Free
Makes 4 servings | 115 calories per serving

2 portobello mushrooms

1 tablespoon olive oil

¼ teaspoon sea salt

1 large bunch arugula, chopped

½ head radicchio, shredded

Dressing

2 tablespoons olive oil

2 tablespoons balsamic vinegar ᴾᵀ, ᴹᴹᴳᶠ

¼ teaspoon dried thyme

¼ teaspoon dried rosemary

¼ teaspoon dried oregano

¼ teaspoon dried sage

¼ cup chopped fresh parsley

1 teaspoon sea salt

1. Preheat the oven to 400°F.
2. Trim the stems off the mushrooms, then lightly rinse the mushrooms and pat dry. Scoop out the gills.
3. Brush the mushrooms on all sides with the olive oil and rub a little salt into them.
4. Place on a baking sheet and roast for 10 minutes. Then turn them over and roast another 10 minutes.
5. Slice the mushrooms and arrange on top of a bed of arugula and radicchio.
6. In a separate bowl, whisk together the dressing ingredients and pour the dressing over the mushrooms and greens.

Notes: Some very nice Italian flavors give these meaty mushrooms a delicious taste, enhanced by the peppery arugula and the bitterness of radicchio. • The color contrast between the three main ingredients is quite striking on the plate. –Chef Philip

Roasted Corn with Cilantro & Lime Zest

Vegan, Gluten-Free, Dairy-Free
Makes 4 servings | 115 calories per serving

Kernels from 4 ears corn

1 teaspoon sea salt

1 tablespoon grapeseed oil

¼ cup chopped fresh cilantro

2 tablespoons chopped fresh sage

2 tablespoons lime zest

2 tablespoons balsamic vinegar [PT, MMGF]

1. Preheat the oven to 425°F.
2. Combine the corn with the salt and oil and place in a roasting pan.
3. Roast, covered, for 30 minutes, or until the corn is slightly caramelized.
4. Transfer the corn to a bowl and add the rest of the ingredients. Stir to combine and serve warm or at room temperature.

Notes: Wonderful Mexican flavors in this delightful summer dish. • Fresh corn is a wonderful treat in the summer, and you can grill the corn cobs on the barbecue instead of roasting for even better flavor. • Include some chopped roasted red peppers (if not a trigger) for added color and texture in this exceptional dish, though it will taste fine without. –Chef Philip

Leafy Green Salad

Vegan, Gluten-Free, Dairy-Free
Makes 4 servings | 132 calories per serving

Dressing

2 tablespoons balsamic vinegar [PT, MMGF]

2 tablespoons olive oil

¼ teaspoon dried thyme

¼ teaspoon dried marjoram or oregano

½ teaspoon mustard powder

¼ teaspoon sea salt

4 cups torn salad greens mixture
   (purslane, leaf lettuce, dandelion
   greens, beet greens, frisée; use a variety of colors and shapes)

1 cucumber, diced

1 carrot, grated

1 raw purple beet, peeled and grated

1 tablespoon toasted sesame seeds [PT]

10 pitted olives, sliced (not oil-cured)

1. Whisk all of the dressing ingredients together in a bowl and pour over the salad greens. Toss to evenly coat the leaves in the dressing. Drain excess dressing.
2. Arrange the vegetables, sesame seeds, and olives decoratively over the salad greens and serve immediately.

Notes: Tear the salad greens by hand instead of cutting them with a knife to prevent discoloring. • A very quick and easy everyday salad with a variety of colors, textures, and flavors. —Chef Philip

Brussels Sprout Slaw

Vegan, Gluten-Free, Dairy-Free
Makes 4 servings | 74 calories per serving

20 Brussels sprouts, shredded

10 fresh basil leaves, chopped

1½ tablespoons toasted sesame oil[PT]

1 tablespoon rice vinegar [PT, MMGF]

2 teaspoons mirin[PT]

1½ tablespoons tamari (gluten-free soy sauce)

1. Toss all of the ingredients in a bowl together and let marinate a half hour before serving.

Notes: A Japanese variation on the classic slaw idea. • Cabbage and/or red cabbage (or a combination of both) can be used as a substitute for the Brussels sprouts. —Chef Philip

Dandelions with Garlic-Oil Dressing

Vegan, Gluten-Free, Dairy-Free
Makes 4 servings | 80 calories per serving

1 large bunch dandelions, chopped

2 tablespoons garlic-infused olive oil[PT] (page 220)

1 teaspoon rice vinegar [PT, MMGF]

½ teaspoon sea salt

1. Blanch the dandelions by dropping them in boiling water for a few seconds. Rinse with cold water, drain, and squeeze out excess water.
2. Place the dandelions in a bowl and add the rest of the ingredients. Toss to combine and let sit for an hour before serving.

Notes: Although often mistaken for a weed, dandelions are a very flavorful bitter green with a high amount of vitamins and minerals. • Dandelions are used widely in many cuisines since they are so incredibly easy to grow. –Sonia

Spinach with Sesame Dressing

Vegan, Gluten-Free, Dairy-Free
Makes 4 servings | 85 calories per serving

1 pound fresh spinach leaves

¼ cup toasted sesame seeds[PT]

1 tablespoon seaweed-mushroom stock (page 218)

1½ tablespoons tamari (gluten-free soy sauce)

1 teaspoon sake[PT]

1 tablespoon mirin[PT]

1. Blanch the spinach by dropping it in boiling water for a few seconds. Then immediately drain it and rinse the spinach under cold water. Squeeze all water out of the spinach and set aside.
2. In a mortar and pestle or a food processor, grind the sesame seeds down.
3. Combine the stock, tamari, sake, mirin, and ground sesame seeds in a bowl.
4. Coat the spinach with the sesame seed dressing.

Notes: This classic sesame seed dressing from Japan works well with a variety of blanched vegetables besides spinach—green beans, shredded collard greens, and rapini, in particular. –Chef Philip

Wilted Kale Salad

Vegan, Gluten-Free, Dairy-Free
Makes 4 servings | 115 calories per serving

1 bunch kale, stalks removed, leaves
  chopped very small
1 tablespoon balsamic vinegar ^{PT, MMGF}
½ teaspoon sea salt
1 carrot, grated

1 tablespoon lemon zest
1 tablespoon toasted pumpkin seeds
1 teaspoon mirin^{PT}
1 tablespoon olive oil

1. Place the kale in a bowl and massage the balsamic vinegar and salt into the kale. Let sit for 30 minutes.
2. Add the rest of the ingredients and mix well to coat the kale leaves.

Notes: Kale has become tremendously popular in recent years due to its versatility, nutritional value, and ease of cultivation. • This is an easy and flavorful dish. –Chef Philip

SIDES

Oat Pilaf

Vegan, Dairy-Free, Detox-Friendly
Makes 4 servings | 200 calories per serving

1 tablespoon olive oil

1 stalk celery, diced

3 cremini, button, or shiitake
  mushrooms, chopped

⅓ cup fresh shelled peas

1 carrot, diced

1 teaspoon sea salt

1 cup whole dried oats^{MMGF}

3 cups water or seaweed-mushroom or
  vegetable stock (pages 217–218)

¼ cup chopped fresh parsley

1. In a saucepan, heat up the olive oil, then add the celery, mushrooms, peas, carrots, and salt and cook for 5 minutes.
2. Add the oats and water and bring to a boil.
3. Lower the heat, cover tightly, and cook for 50 minutes. Garnish with the parsley.

Notes: Whole oats have a creamy, delightful texture and are eaten often in Scotland. • If you like the creaminess of oatmeal, please try this pilaf for a new side dish instead of rice or other grains. —Chef Philip

Quinoa Pilaf

Vegan, Gluten-Free, Dairy-Free
Makes 4 servings | 240 calories per serving

1 teaspoon olive oil

1 stalk celery, diced

1 small carrot, diced

1 cup quinoa

1 teaspoon sea salt

2 cups boiling water or vegetable stock
(page 217)

2 tablespoons chopped fresh parsley

¼ cup raisins[PT]

2 tablespoons pine nuts

1. Heat up a pot over medium heat and add the olive oil, celery, and carrot and cook for 2 minutes, stirring regularly.
2. Add the quinoa. Stirring constantly, cook 1 minute, or until you smell a nutty aroma.
3. Add the sea salt and boiling water.
4. Bring to a simmer, cover, lower the heat, and cook for 20 minutes.
5. Remove from the heat and add the parsley, raisins, and pine nuts. Stir gently to combine.

Notes: Quinoa is the only grain that is a complete protein, thus making it one of the most nutritious grains. • The Incan empire was raised on this lovely grain, which has recently gained popularity in the United States and Europe due to its appealing nutty flavor. • Quinoa is very light in texture, making it more popular in summer than in winter. • Quinoa comes in three colors: red, black, and white; white is the most popular. • For added color in this dish, use all three colors of quinoa. –Chef Philip

Roasted Eggplant

Vegan, Gluten-Free, Dairy-Free, Detox-Friendly
Makes 4 servings | 65 calories per serving

1 small eggplant

1 teaspoon sea salt

1 tablespoon olive oil

1. Cut the eggplant into ½-inch-thick slices.
2. Sprinkle the salt on the eggplant slices and massage it in gently.
3. Put the eggplant in a colander set over a bowl to drain for 1 hour.
4. Preheat the oven to 425°F.
5. Brush the eggplant slices with the olive oil.
6. Roast in a single layer on a baking sheet for 15 minutes. Then turn over and roast another 10 minutes, or until the eggplant is slightly charred.

Notes: This is a stand-alone side dish and goes very well with the Hummus Salad (page 129). • You can sprinkle the eggplant slices with dried spices such as rosemary, oregano, or sumac before roasting. –Chef Philip

Anadama Bread

Vegan, Dairy-Free, Detox-Friendly
Makes 2 loaves | 95 calories per serving

1 teaspoon dry yeast^NGF

2 tablespoons blackstrap molasses

1 cup warm water (100°F)

1 cup soymilk

2 teaspoons sea salt

2 cups cornmeal^MMGF

2 cups white flour^NGF

Olive oil, for brushing

1. Add the yeast and blackstrap molasses to the warm water in a bowl and whisk.
2. Let sit for 5 minutes, until foamy.
3. Add the soymilk and sea salt and whisk together.
4. Slowly start to incorporate first the cornmeal and then the flour into the yeast mixture. At first with a spoon, and then laying the dough on a flat surface and using your hands, knead the dough for 10 minutes, until smooth and shiny. Add more flour if it gets too sticky.
5. Brush the dough with olive oil, place in a bowl, and cover with a towel. Let sit about 1 hour, or until the dough has doubled in size.
6. Cut the dough in half, shape into loaves, and place on an oiled baking sheet or into oiled loaf pans. Cover and let rise another hour, or until doubled in size.
7. Preheat the oven to 500°F.
8. Bake loaves for 25 minutes, or until golden brown.

Notes: This is a personal favorite bread of mine; I started making this bread back in graduate school. • This recipe comes from the northeastern United States and is one of the first culinary fusions of the clash of two worlds when the Native Americans first encountered the pilgrims • The combination of corn and wheat provides wonderful flavor and texture, slightly sweetened and darkened by the molasses. • Traditionally made with cow's milk, this vegan version uses soymilk, though I have also used hemp milk and almond milk, both providing different, equally interesting tastes. –Chef Philip

Salmon Fried Rice

Gluten-Free, Dairy-Free
Makes 4 servings | 375 calories per serving

¼ cup olive oil

8 ounces smoked salmon

¼ cup fresh shelled peas

¼ cup diced carrots, ¼-inch pieces

3 egg whites

1 egg yolk

3 cups cooked rice

Salt to taste

1. Heat the oil in a pan over medium-high, then add the smoked salmon and sauté until cooked through, breaking it into bite-size pieces with a spatula while stir-frying.
2. Add the peas and carrots and cook until the carrots start to soften.
3. Whisk the egg whites and egg yolk together, then add to the pan. Scramble until cooked through.
4. Add the rice and mix well. Cook until the rice is heated through.
5. Season with salt to taste.

Notes: Have leftover rice and don't know what to do with it? Use it here. • This is a simple and quick dish that's made healthier with the addition of salmon, which contains a lot of healthy fat. –Sonia

Fennel Roasted Beets

Vegan, Gluten-Free, Dairy-Free
Makes 4 servings | 60 calories per serving

1 large purple beet, peeled and diced

1 small bulb fresh fennel, diced

1 tablespoon grapeseed oil

1 teaspoon sea salt

1 tablespoon balsamic vinegar [PT, MMGF]

1. Preheat the oven to 425°F.
2. Place the diced beets and diced fennel in a roasting pan with the oil and salt. Stir to coat well. Cover and roast for 30 minutes, or until slightly browned and caramelized on the edges.
3. Toss with the balsamic vinegar and serve.

Notes: A classic combination of fennel and beets is a favorite from Eastern Europe. • The beautiful color of the beets with the sweet licorice flavor of the fennel works in any season and brightens up any plate! • Fennel is very good for reflux. —Chef Philip

Rustic Whole-Wheat Bread

Vegan, Dairy-Free, Detox-Friendly
Makes 2 loaves | 100 calories per slice

1 teaspoon dry yeast[NGF]

1 tablespoon agave

2 cups warm water (100°F)

2 teaspoons sea salt

2 cups white flour[NGF]

2 cups whole-wheat flour[NGF]

1 tablespoon olive oil

1. Add the yeast and agave to the warm water in a bowl and whisk.
2. Let sit 5 minutes, until foamy.
3. Add the sea salt and whisk.
4. Slowly start to incorporate the flours into the yeast mixture. At first with a spoon, and then laying the dough on a flat surface and using your hands, knead the dough for 10 minutes, until smooth and shiny. Add more flour if it gets too sticky.
5. Brush the dough with the olive oil, place in a bowl, and cover with a towel. Let sit about 1 hour, or until the dough has doubled in size.
6. Cut the dough in half, shape into loaves, and place on an oiled baking sheet or into oiled loaf pans. Cover and let rise another hour, or until doubled in size.
7. Preheat the oven to 500°F.
8. Bake the loaves for 25 minutes, or until golden brown.

Notes: If you have never baked bread before, this is a good basic recipe to start with. • Please look at videos online to learn the basics of kneading and rising. • Baking bread is a very meditative practice for many people, including those who do not otherwise cook. —Chef Philip

Stir-Fried Brussels Sprouts

Vegan, Gluten-Free, Dairy-Free
Makes 4 servings | 60 calories per serving

About 20 Brussels sprouts

1 teaspoon sesame oil[PT]

1 tablespoon minced fresh ginger

1 tablespoon tamari (gluten-free soy sauce)

1 tablespoon mirin[PT]

1 tablespoon sake[PT]

1 teaspoon toasted sesame oil[PT]

Cooked brown rice, for serving

1. Trim the bottom ends off the sprouts and then thinly slice.
2. In a hot wok or frying pan, add the sesame oil and ginger and stir-fry for 30 seconds.
3. Add the sprouts and stir-fry for 5 minutes.
4. Add the tamari, mirin, and sake and stir-fry for 1 minute.
5. Remove from the heat, add the toasted sesame oil, and stir well. Serve with brown rice.

Notes: If possible, purchase Brussels sprouts that are still on the stalk for ultimate freshness and flavor. • Usually Brussels sprouts are cooked whole or halved, whereas in this recipe we are slicing them thinly for a different texture.
—Chef Philip

Rice with Cumin & Turmeric

Vegan, Gluten-Free, Dairy-Free, Detox-Friendly
Makes 4 servings | 200 calories per serving

1. Add all of the ingredients to a rice cooker and cook according to the manu-

1 cup uncooked rice

2 cups vegetable stock (page 217)

1 tablespoon olive oil

1 teaspoon sea salt

½ teaspoon ground cumin

½ teaspoon ground turmeric

facturer's instructions.
2. Fluff the rice with a fork and serve immediately.

Notes: Use a rice cooker for this recipe. If you don't have one, they're relatively inexpensive. • This rice dish is a beautiful golden color and goes great with almost everything, especially fish. • I use jasmine rice because it isn't sticky, and my preferred ratio of liquid to rice is 3:2. • This is a staple in my house. • This recipe is so good, I have taken it straight from my previous book, Dropping Acid: The Reflux Cookbook & Cure. *–Dr. Jamie*

Cold Noodles with Sesame Sauce

Vegan, Dairy-Free
Makes 4 servings | 500 calories per serving

1. Boil the noodles until cooked, drain, rinse with cold water, and drain again.

1 pound ramen noodles[NGF] (or other type of Chinese noodle or soba noodles)

2 cucumbers (preferably Japanese or Persian), shredded

1 large carrot, julienned

Sauce

⅓ cup tamari (gluten-free soy sauce)

¼ cup mirin[PT]

2 tablespoons rice vinegar [PT, MMGF]

1 tablespoon chinkiang vinegar [PT, MMGF]

¼ cup tahini[PT]

2 tablespoons toasted sesame oil[PT]

Place in a bowl and top with the cucumber and carrot.

2. Place all of the sauce ingredients in a blender and blend until smooth, adding water or stock if needed to thin it out.

3. Season the sauce to taste with more tamari or vinegar and serve over the noodles and vegetables.

Notes: This is a famous dish found all over China, with variations from region to region. • Very refreshing on a hot summer day or evening. • If chili peppers or chili oil is not a trigger, please add for more flavor, as the chilies will help cool you down along with the cucumber and cold noodles. –Sonia

Emperor's Jade Fried Rice
Vegetarian, Gluten-Free, Dairy-Free

1. Heat 2 tablespoons of the oil in a pan over medium-high heat, then add the spinach and mustard greens and sauté until wilted. Remove from the heat

4 tablespoons olive oil

2 cups chopped spinach

2 cups chopped mustard greens

3 egg whites

1 egg yolk

4 cups cooked rice

¼ cup diced smoked tofu (see page 179), ¼-inch pieces

Salt to taste

and drain the excess water from the pan.

2. Remove the greens from the pan and set aside.
3. Heat the remaining 2 tablespoons oil in the same pan over medium-high heat. Whisk the egg whites and egg yolk together, then add to the pan. Scramble the eggs until cooked through.
4. Add the rice, spinach and mustard greens mixture, and smoked tofu and mix well. Cook until heated through.
5. Season with salt to taste.

Notes: This recipe is a great way to use up leftover rice. In fact, day-old rice works much better in any fried rice recipes. • This dish is usually made with other leftover ingredients as well, an everything-but-the-kitchen-sink approach. • Here we use chopped spinach to give it an interesting jade green color. –Sonia

Cold Somen Noodles

with Dipping Sauce

Vegan, Dairy-Free
Makes 4 servings | 460 calories per serving

1. Place all of the sauce ingredients in a saucepan. Bring to a boil, lower the

Dipping sauce

1⅔ cups seaweed-mushroom stock (page 218)

½ cup sake[PT]

¼ cup tamari (gluten-free soy sauce)

½ teaspoon salt

½ teaspoon palm sugar

1 pound somen noodles[NGF] or angel hair pasta[NGF]

Several ice cubes

1 sheet nori, cut into thin shreds

2 teaspoons prepared wasabi[MMGF]

   heat, and simmer for 3 minutes. Chill completely.

2. Cook the noodles according to the package directions. Drain under cold water until cool, then drain again.

3. To serve, place a couple cubes of ice into individual serving bowls. Place noodles over ice. Each person gets another bowl for the sauce.

4. Garnish the noodles with nori and wasabi.

5. To eat, take the noodles, dip in the sauce, and slurp away!

Notes: Another wonderful, delicate cold noodle recipe for summer, this comes from Japan and is particularly popular with women, thus sometimes considered a feminine dish. • Somen noodles are very thin wheat noodles, found in Japanese and most Asian markets. —Chef Philip

Sweet Potatoes, Cabbage & Kale

1. Steam the sweet potatoes and kale for 10 minutes, or until cooked.

1 large sweet potato, peeled and chopped into 1-inch cubes	½ head purple cabbage, chopped
1 bunch kale, stalks removed, leaves chopped	2 tablespoons tamari (gluten-free soy sauce)
2 tablespoons olive oil	1 tablespoon palm sugar
3 tablespoons grated fresh ginger	¼ cup chopped fresh cilantro, for garnish

2. In a hot frying pan, add the olive oil.
3. Add the ginger and sauté for 2 minutes.
4. Add the purple cabbage and sauté for 10 minutes.
5. Add the steamed sweet potatoes and kale, tamari, and palm sugar. Cook until heated through.
6. Garnish with the cilantro.

Notes: This is a gorgeous, colorful dish that will brighten up your plate and your day! • Three very different vegetables come together, accented by ginger. • Serve with tempeh or Tofu Cutlets (page 175). –Chef Philip

Yummy Roasted Mashed Root Vegetables

Vegan, Gluten-Free, Dairy-Free, Detox-Friendly
Makes 4 servings | 130 calories per serving

1. Preheat the oven to 425°F.

2 small potatoes, peeled and cut into
  1-inch cubes

1 large parsnip, peeled and cut into
  1-inch cubes

1 medium-size sweet potato (preferably
  satsuma imo), peeled and cut into
  1-inch cubes

1 small celery root, peeled and cut into
  1-inch cubes

1 tablespoon grapeseed oil

1 teaspoon sea salt

¼ cup chopped fresh parsley, for
  garnish

2. Toss the vegetables with the oil and salt and place in a roasting pan. Cover
   with foil and roast for 40 minutes, or until slightly caramelized.
3. Mash the roasted vegetables with a fork or a potato masher.
4. Garnish with the chopped parsley.

*Notes: If you love mashed potatoes you will really love this dish, as it is a glorified
version, enhanced with the flavors of other root vegetables. —Chef Philip*

Stir-Fried Green Beans with Ginger

Vegan, Dairy-Free

1. Bring the water and baking soda to a rapid boil in a pot over high heat.
2. Drop the green beans in the boiling water for 5 seconds to blanch them.

1 quart water	1 tablespoon shaoshing wine [PT, MMGF]
⅛ teaspoon baking soda[MMGF]	1 teaspoon palm sugar
1 pound Chinese long beans or string beans (remove the strings if using string beans)	1 tablespoon sesame oil[PT]
	1 teaspoon fermented black beans[NGF,PT]
	3 tablespoons minced fresh ginger

   Immediately drain and rinse under cold water to stop the cooking process.
3. In a bowl, combine the shaoshing with the tamari and palm sugar and set aside.
4. In a hot wok or frying pan over medium-high heat, add the sesame oil, fermented black beans, and ginger and stir-fry for 2 minutes.
5. Add the blanched beans and stir-fry another 2 minutes.
6. Add the shaoshing mixture and cook for 10 seconds, stirring to coat.

Notes: From China, a delightful summer and fall dish, when fresh green beans are available. • There are many variations on this dish, often including garlic and fermented mustard greens. • This is a simple version flavored with ginger and fermented black beans. –Chef Philip

Carrots with Mustard Seeds & Raisins
Vegan, Gluten-Free, Dairy-Free

Makes 4 servings | 95 calories per serving

1 tablespoon olive oil

2 teaspoons black mustard seeds[MMGF]

4 large carrots, grated

¼ cup raisins[PT]

1. In a hot wok or frying pan over medium-high heat, add the olive oil.
2. Add the mustard seeds and cook a few seconds, or until they start to pop.
3. Remove from the heat and add the carrots, stirring to coat the carrots with the seeds and oil.
4. Add the raisins and serve.

Notes: Another very fast, easy to produce, and inexpensive dish with very flavorful results. –Chef Philip

Stir-Fried Corn with Miso & Basil

Vegan, Gluten-Free, Dairy-Free
Makes 4 servings | 125 calories per serving

1 tablespoon olive oil

Kernels from 4 ears corn

2 tablespoons white miso

2 tablespoons sake[PT]

1 tablespoon mirin[PT]

2 tablespoons vegetable or seaweed-
mushroom stock (page 218)

½ cup chopped fresh basil

1. In a hot wok or frying pan over medium-high heat, add the olive oil and corn and stir-fry for 3 minutes.
2. In a separate bowl, combine the miso, sake, mirin, and stock.
3. Add the miso mixture to the wok and stir-fry until it starts to bubble and thicken. Remove from the heat, add the basil, and serve hot.

Notes: Although corn is an ingredient native to North and Central America, it has found its way into many culinary traditions since the 16th century. • Due to its wonderful flavor, simplicity in growing, and high nutrition, corn has been accepted all over the world and can be found in markets on every continent. • I came up with this dish while visiting Tokyo one fall; preparing a very American ingredient with some very typical Japanese ingredients made for a wonderful and unexpected result. –Chef Philip

Pickled Bean Sprouts

Vegan, Gluten-Free, Dairy-Free
Makes 4 servings | 45 calories per serving

3 cups water

⅛ teaspoon baking soda^{MMGF}

1 pound mung bean or soybean
  sprouts

2 tablespoons tamari (gluten-free soy
  sauce)

1 tablespoon mirin^{PT}

1 tablespoon rice vinegar ^{PT, MMGF}

1. Bring the water and baking soda to a boil in a pot over medium-high heat.
2. Blanch the sprouts by dropping them in the boiling water and then immediately removing them.
3. Immediately rinse under cold water to stop the cooking process. Drain and transfer the sprouts to a bowl.
4. Add the tamari, mirin, and rice vinegar to the blanched sprouts and let marinate for 2 hours before serving.

Notes: A very simple Japanese and Chinese approach to preparing bean sprouts.
• This dish can be refrigerated for up to 3 days and can be used as a side dish with any kind of Asian-inspired meal. • If you like sprouts, you may want to consider getting your own sprouting jar to grow your own. —Chef Philip

Taiwanese Dill with Ginger

Vegan, Gluten-Free, Dairy-Free
Makes 4 servings | 100 calories per serving

3 tablespoons olive oil

2 (¼-inch-thick) slices fresh ginger
 (no need to peel)

1 bunch dill, chopped (about 3–4 cups)

1 tablespoon rice wine^PT

¼ cup water or seaweed-mushroom or
 vegetable stock (pages 217–218)

Salt to taste

1. Heat the oil in a pan over medium-high heat, then add the ginger and sauté until fragrant, about 1 minute.
2. Add the dill, rice wine, water, and salt to taste and cook for 2–3 minutes. Serve hot.

Notes: Although dill is an herb, in this case it's used as a vegetable. • It is frequently served in Taiwan as a fragrant side dish over rice. –Sonia

Roasted Butternut Squash Purée

Vegan, Gluten-Free, Dairy-Free, Detox-Friendly
Makes 4 servings | 90 calories per serving

1 butternut squash, peeled, seeded, and diced

1 tablespoon grapeseed oil

1 teaspoon sea salt

1. Preheat the oven to 425°F.
2. Combine the squash, grapeseed oil, and salt in a roasting pan and mix until the squash is well coated.
3. Cover with foil and roast for 30 minutes.
4. Mash squash with a fork or a potato masher, or purée in a food processor.

Notes: In fall and winter, pumpkins and squashes are all over my kitchen and menus. • This Native American ingredient is packed with flavor and nutrition and can be used in so many recipes, from soups to desserts. • I frequently host multiple-course pumpkin menus at the underground restaurant every winter to celebrate one of the greatest vegetables. • For variations on this recipe, add ½ teaspoon cinnamon to the purée, or add some chopped dried fruit and chopped pistachios. —Chef Philip

Roasted Asparagus with Black Olives

Vegan, Gluten-Free, Dairy-Free
Makes 4 servings | 155 calories per serving

1 pound asparagus, 2 inches trimmed off bottoms

¼ cup pitted and chopped black olives[PT]

2 tablespoons chopped fresh parsley

2 tablespoons white wine[PT]

1 tablespoon olive oil

1. Preheat the oven to 425°F.
2. Combine all of the ingredients in a bowl and mix well.
3. Place on a baking sheet in a single layer and roast, uncovered, for 15 minutes, or until asparagus is tender.

Notes: In late winter and early spring, when asparagus starts to come into season, this remarkable vegetable makes many appearances in my kitchen. • This is an easily prepared Italian spring side dish that goes very well with Tempeh Marsala (page 174) or any other Italian or Mediterranean entrée. —Chef Philip

Polenta with Pistachios & Fennel

Vegan, Gluten-Free, Dairy-Free
Makes 4 servings | 325 calories per serving

2 tablespoons olive oil

⅓ cup minced fennel bulb, ⅛-inch pieces

1½ teaspoons sea salt

1 cup polenta

½ cup raw pistachios[PT]

2 cups soymilk

2 cups seaweed-mushroom stock
 (page 218)

2 tablespoons chopped fresh parsley

1 tablespoon chopped fresh basil

1. In a saucepan, add the olive oil, fennel, and sea salt and sauté for 4 minutes over medium heat.
2. Add the polenta, pistachios, soymilk, and stock and bring to a simmer over high heat.
3. Lower the heat and continue cooking for 30 minutes, stirring regularly. The polenta will thicken, so you must stir to keep it from sticking.
4. Add the parsley and basil.
5. Remove from the heat and pour the polenta into an oiled baking dish.
6. Let cool and set for 2 hours.
7. Cut pieces of polenta and eat as is or grill before serving.

Notes: Polenta is one of the great ways of enjoying the goodness of corn when not in season. • Although native to North and Central America, corn has found its way into many cuisines since the 16th century. • In Italy, corn is dried to a course meal and thus enjoyed in breads and as polenta all year long. –Chef Philip

Korean Cold Noodles with Soy-Sesame Milk (Kong gook soo)

Vegan, Dairy-Free
Makes 4 servings | 315 calories per serving

1 cup dried soybeans

¼ cup raw sesame seeds[PT]

1 pound Korean or Japanese soba noodles[NGF]

Several ice cubes

Salt to taste

Daikon sprouts (kaiware), for garnish

1 cucumber, shredded

1. Soak the soybeans and sesame seeds in 2 quarts water overnight or for 8 hours.
2. Drain and rinse the soybeans and sesame seeds and place in a blender with 1 quart cold water. Purée until smooth. Chill until ice cold.
3. Cook the soba noodles according to the package directions. Drain and rinse under cold water until cool, then drain again.
4. Divide the soba among 4 bowls, then pour the cold soy-sesame mixture over each bowl. Add ice to each bowl.
5. Salt to taste.
6. Garnish with daikon sprouts and cucumber.

Notes: A delightful summer dish, incredibly refreshing. This is one of many cold noodle dishes from the unique culinary tradition of Korea. • I learned this dish from my favorite Korean restaurant in Oakland, Pyung Chong Tofu House, a wonderful, small restaurant where everything is handmade, including some amazing noodles to prepare this dish. –Chef Philip

ENTRÉES

Turkey & Mushrooms with Rice

Gluten-Free, Dairy-Free
Makes 6 servings | 445 calories per serving

6 dried shiitake mushrooms

3 tablespoons olive oil

1 tablespoon minced fresh ginger

1 pound ground turkey

½ cup rice wine[PT]

½ cup tamari (gluten-free soy sauce)

2 cups water

1 teaspoon sugar

½ teaspoon Chinese spice blend
 (page 220)

1 star anise

Cooked rice, for serving

Chopped fresh cilantro, for garnish

Julienned carrots, for garnish

Bean sprouts, for garnish

1. In warm water, soak the mushrooms until soft. Rinse the mushrooms and pat dry. Remove the stems and thinly slice the caps.
2. Heat the oil in a pan over medium-high heat. Add the ginger and sauté for 1 minute. Add the mushrooms and turkey and sauté until the turkey is browned.
3. Add the wine, tamari, water, sugar, Chinese spice blend, and star anise. Bring to a boil, then lower the heat to simmer for 45 minutes.
4. Remove the star anise and discard. Serve over rice and garnish with cilantro, carrots, and bean sprouts.

Notes: A variation of this comfort food is sold on the streets all over Taiwan, and every family has a slightly different version of this dish. • I tend to use the low-fat ground turkey meat instead of traditional ground pork. • The vegetable garnish adds a crunchy freshness to the dish. —Sonia

One-Pot Ginger Chicken Rice

Gluten-Free, Dairy-Free
Makes 4 servings | 675 calories per serving

Marinated chicken

⅛ teaspoon salt

2 tablespoons tamari (gluten-free soy sauce)

2 tablespoons olive oil

2 tablespoons rice wine[PT]

4 chicken breasts

6 dried shiitake or portobello mushrooms

3 tablespoons olive oil

12 (⅛-inch-thick) slices peeled fresh ginger

2 cups uncooked jasmine or other long grain rice 1½ cups chicken stock (page 217)

¼ cup rice wine[PT] (preferably shaoshing [PT, MMGF])

Sea salt to taste

1–2 tablespoons tamari (gluten-free soy sauce)

Few dashes of sesame oil[PT]

Chopped fresh cilantro, for garnish

1. For the marinated chicken, mix the salt, tamari, olive oil, and rice wine in a large bowl. Add the chicken breasts and marinate the chicken for 30 minutes in the refrigerator. Drain and set aside the chicken (discard the marinade).
2. In warm water, soak the mushrooms until soft. Rinse the mushrooms and pat dry. Remove the stems and thinly slice the caps.
3. Heat the oil in a pan over medium-high heat and sauté the ginger until fragrant for 1 minute.
4. Add the rice and mix well to coat with oil.
5. Add the chicken stock, rice wine, and salt to taste and mix well.
6. Transfer to a rice cooker and place the chicken breasts and mushrooms on top. Cook the rice according to the manufacturer's instructions. (Alternatively, if you don't have a rice cooker, cook in a pot on the stovetop for at least 20–25 minutes.)
7. Once the rice and chicken are cooked, let stand for 10 minutes, covered.

8. Meanwhile, mix the tamari and sesame oil in a serving bowl.

9. Garnish the rice and chicken with cilantro and serve with the sauce.

Notes: Put everything in a rice cooker and voila! What a very simple dish to make. • My mother would always make this using a rice cooker; however, it can be made on the stovetop in a pot (following the rice cooking directions on the package) in about 20–25 minutes. • Mom would add Chinese sausage to the mix for extra flavor. Here we omit the sausage for a healthier version. • Sesame oil may be a trigger food for some people. • Serve with Taiwanese Dill with Ginger (page 161) or other sautéed greens. –Sonia

Ginger Tempeh

Vegan, Gluten-Free, Dairy-Free
Makes 4 servings | 180 calories per serving

2 teaspoons cornstarch,[MMGF] potato starch, or kudzu ½ cup vegetable stock (page 217)

½ pound tempeh, cut into ½-inch strips

2 tablespoons tamari (gluten-free soy sauce)

1 tablespoon shaoshing wine[PT, MMGF] or dry sherry[PT]

1 tablespoon mirin[PT]

1 tablespoon grapeseed oil

2 tablespoons chopped fresh ginger

1 small head broccoli, cut into small florets

2 tablespoons chopped fresh cilantro or basil, for garnish

Cooked brown rice, for serving

1. Preheat the oven to 400°F.
2. Dissolve the cornstarch in the stock and set aside.
3. Place the tempeh on an oiled baking sheet and bake for 20 minutes, or until lightly browned. Set aside.
4. In a bowl, mix the tamari, shaoshing, and mirin and set aside.
5. In a hot wok or frying pan over medium-high heat, add the grapeseed oil.
6. Add the ginger and stir-fry for 30 seconds.
7. Add the broccoli and stir-fry for 3 minutes, or until the vegetable is bright green and slightly soft.
8. Add the tamari mixture and stir-fry for 10 more seconds.
9. Add the dissolved cornstarch and stock and stir-fry for 30 seconds, until it bubbles and thickens.
10. Add the tempeh and stir to coat, cooking until warmed through.
11. Garnish with the cilantro and serve with brown rice.

Notes: Close call here: the shaoshing and sherry might be labeled as possible triggers, but the amount called for is small enough that this dish might be detox-friendly. • Such a flavorful dish! • The warming effect of ginger makes this an ideal winter or cold fall evening dish. • Very nice to serve with rice and seaweed salad. • It is worth seeking out a local tempeh maker/provider, if possible. • I use tempeh in a wide variety of Southeast Asian as well as Italian dishes for its flavor and texture. —Chef Philip

Tuscan-Style White Pork with Rosemary

Gluten-Free
Makes 6 servings | 285 calories per serving

2 small- to medium-size pork tenderloins

1 teaspoon sea salt

2–3 tablespoons olive oil

1 large bunch fresh rosemary, or 2 handfuls

1–1½ quarts low-fat milk

1. Cut each of the pork tenderloins into three pieces and salt all sides.
2. Heat the oil in a soup pot over medium-high and brown the 6 pork pieces.
3. When the pork pieces are browned, lower the heat to medium and add the rosemary.
4. Cover the rosemary and the meat with milk; this will take about a quart, possibly more.
5. Bring to a slow bubbling boil and cook for 45 minutes.
6. Remove the meat and slice, serving each portion with some of the intact rosemary stems.

Notes: This really easy and yummy dish was given to me by my friend Dora. • This dish makes the entire house smell wonderful because of the rosemary. • And yes, this dish requires fresh rosemary; dried will not do. • Serve with Yummy Roasted Mashed Root Vegetables (page 156) and sautéed string beans or Roasted Asparagus with Black Olives (page 163) • I no longer eat dairy, but I used to adore this recipe; unfortunately, it doesn't work with almond milk. Oh well. –Dr. Jamie

Tempeh Marsala

Vegan, Dairy-Free
Makes 4 servings | 340 calories per serving

Tempeh

Bowl one: ½ cup white flour[NGF] mixed with ¼ teaspoon salt

Bowl two: ½ cup soymilk mixed with ¼ teaspoon salt

Bowl three: ½ cup cornmeal[MMGF] mixed with ½ teaspoon salt, ½ teaspoon
dried oregano, ½ teaspoon dried rosemary, ½ teaspoon dried thyme, and
2 tablespoons nutritional yeast

1 pound tempeh, cut into 8 equal-size cutlets

Marsala

2 tablespoons olive oil

¼ pound cremini mushrooms, thinly
sliced

1 cup fresh shelled peas

1 teaspoon dried oregano

1½ teaspoons sea salt

½ cup Marsala wine[PT]

½ teaspoon black pepper[PT] (optional)

¼ cup chopped fresh basil

Directions for the Tempeh

1. Preheat the oven to 425°F.
2. Place the 3 bowls in order in a row.
3. Dip a tempeh cutlet once in the flour (bowl one), flip, and dip the other side.
4. Now dip the same cutlet in the soymilk mixture (bowl two), coating both
   sides, and then dip it in the cornmeal mixture (bowl three), coating both sides.
5. Place the breaded tempeh on a baking sheet lightly coated with oil and
   repeat with the remaining cutlets.
6. Bake for 30 minutes, or until crisp. (Alternatively, deep-fry until golden
   brown.)

Directions for the Marsala

1. In a frying pan, heat up the olive oil.
2. Add the mushrooms, peas, oregano, and salt and cook for 5 minutes.
3. Add the Marsala wine, cover, and cook for another 5 minutes, until the
   alcohol evaporates.
4. Pour over the cutlets.

5. Season with salt and pepper and garnish with basil.

Notes: This is a flavorful vegan version of the classic Italian dish scaloppini, which is usually made with chicken or veal. • Serve with a grain pilaf or risotto and a green salad for a wonderful meal. –Chef Philip

Tofu Cutlets

Vegan, Gluten-Free, Dairy-Free, Detox-Friendly
Makes 4 servings | 160 calories per serving

1. Preheat the oven to 400°F.

1 pound firm tofu, cut into ½-inch-thick slabs

¼ cup cornmeal[MMGF]

¼ cup nutritional yeast

1 teaspoon sea salt

2 tablespoons dried herbs (combination of marjoram, oregano, thyme, basil, sage, rosemary)

⅓ cup soymilk or almond milk

2 tablespoons olive oil

2. Press the tofu by placing the slabs on a towel. Cover with another towel and place a cutting board on the top towel. Place a can or something heavy on the board and let sit for 15 minutes.
3. In a bowl, combine the cornmeal, nutritional yeast, salt, and herbs. Pour the soymilk into a separate bowl.
4. Oil a baking sheet with the olive oil.
5. Dip each piece of tofu in the soymilk and then in the herb-cornmeal mixture, thoroughly coating all sides of each.
6. Place each crusted piece of tofu on the baking sheet, not letting the pieces touch.
7. Bake for 30 minutes, or until nice and crispy.

Notes: Vary the herbs for a variety of flavors in this dish. • These are easy to make and have a nice flavor and texture. • You can also substitute tempeh for the tofu! –Chef Philip

Basil Chicken

Gluten-Free, Dairy-Free
Makes 6 servings | 325 calories per serving

¼ cup sesame oil^{PT} or extra-virgin olive oil

10 (⅛-inch-thick) slices peeled fresh ginger

2 pounds chicken breast, chopped into bite-size chunks 1 cup rice wine^{PT} preferably shaoshing ^{PT, MMGF} or dry sherry^{PT})

1 cup tamari (gluten-free soy sauce)

2 whole star anise, or 1 tablespoon aniseed

1 tablespoon honey

1 bunch fresh basil, chopped

Steamed white rice, for serving

1. Heat the oil in a pan over medium-high heat, then add the ginger and cook until fragrant, about 1 minute.
2. Add the chicken pieces and brown for 1–2 minutes.
3. Add the rice wine, tamari, star anise, and honey and bring to a boil, then reduce the heat to a simmer and cook for 15 minutes, or until the chicken is cooked through.
4. Stir in the basil and remove from the heat. Serve over rice.

Notes: This is a traditional Taiwanese dish that is often called "three cup chicken," with tremendous variations from family to family. • The "three cup" refers to the fact that this dish is usually made with equal parts of rice wine, soy sauce, and sesame oil. —Sonia

Poached Halibut with Prosciutto

Gluten-Free, Dairy-Free
Makes 4 servings | 385 calories per serving

1. Marinate the halibut in the salt and rice wine for 10 minutes.

1 pound halibut, cut into 4 equal-size pieces	4 (⅛-inch-thick) slices peeled fresh ginger
½ teaspoon salt	10 thin slices prosciutto,PT chopped
½ teaspoon rice winePT	10 slices canned bamboo shoots
5 dried shiitake mushrooms	1 cup chicken stock (page 217)
¼ cup olive oil	2–4 tablespoons chopped fresh cilantro, for garnish

2. Soak the mushrooms in warm water until soft. Rinse the mushrooms and pat dry. Remove the stems and thinly slice the caps.
3. Heat the oil in a pan over medium-high heat, then add the ginger and sauté for 1 minute.
4. Add the mushrooms, prosciutto, and bamboo shoots and sauté for 1 minute.
5. Add the halibut and chicken stock and cover the pan.
6. Poach until the fish is cooked through (poach 10–15 minutes per 1 inch of thickness).
7. Top with cilantro and serve.

Notes: The saltiness of the prosciutto and earthiness of the shiitake mushrooms add complexity to this flavorful dish. • This dish is great with steamed rice or the rice dish on page 151. –Sonia

Steamed Mussels & Shrimp Pot

Gluten-Free, Dairy-Free
Makes 3–4 servings | 450 calories per serving

1. Place your biggest stockpot with a lid (one that will hold all of the ingredi-

3–4 tablespoons olive oil

½ teaspoon sea salt

2 shallots,^{PT} diced

1 bulb fennel (not the green parts), coarsely chopped

1–2 large tomatoes,^{PT} diced

1–2 cups chicken stock (page 217); enough to cover the bottom of your pot, ½ to 1 inch up the side)

4 pounds fresh mussels, scrubbed and debearded

1–1½ pounds fresh uncooked shrimp, shell on

¼ cup chopped fresh cilantro leaves, for garnish

ents) over medium-high heat and add the olive oil. Then add the salt, shallots, and fennel. Sauté until soft.
2. Add the tomato and continue to cook.
3. Add the chicken stock and bring to a boil over high heat.
4. When the stock is boiling, add the mussels and shrimp and cover.
5. Every 2–3 minutes, with a large serving utensil, move the mussels and shrimp about so that the bottom ones come to the top.
6. When all of the mussels have opened (discard any that haven't), after about 10–12 minutes of steaming, garnish with cilantro and serve in big bowls.

Notes: This recipe comes with a warning: if shallots or tomatoes are trigger foods for your reflux, you may need to consider leaving them out. • In truth, the fennel, chicken stock, and cilantro are enough to add great flavor to the "sauce." • This recipe is wonderful in the summer when all of the ingredients are fresh. • People go gaga for this dish, and the bread eaters can have at the sauce with wild aban-don. • This can be a messy meal; I recommend that you eat out on the deck, and put newspaper down on the table! • Fennel is a good-for-reflux food, and you can add it to lots of recipes in this book; it is great with just about any salad. • I also like roasting fennel on the grill, just as another veggie. –Dr. Jamie

Four-Star Marinated Smoked Tempeh

Vegan, Gluten-Free, Dairy-Free
Makes 4 servings | 275 calories per serving

2 tablespoons tamari (gluten-free soy sauce)

1 tablespoon sesame oil^{PT}

1 tablespoon mirin^{PT}

1 tablespoon maple syrup

2 tablespoons seaweed-mushroom stock (page 218)

1 pound tempeh (usually this will be two ½-pound packages)

Apple wood or cherry wood, for smoking

1. Mix together all of the ingredients (except the tempeh and apple wood) in a bowl. Add the tempeh and let marinate for 1 hour.
2. Smoke over apple wood or cherry wood for about 15 minutes, or until browned and aromatic.

Notes: We can also smoke tofu with the same method. • Use firm tofu that has been cut into ½-inch-thick slabs and pressed for 15 minutes before marinating for 1 hour. • To smoke the tempeh on a stovetop smoker: Place the wood chips on the bottom of smoker. Place the drip tray on top of chips. Place the smoking tray on top of drip tray. Place the tempeh on smoking tray, cover tightly with lid, and put on the stove over medium heat. Check at 15 minutes. Always have your exhaust fans on high when using a stovetop smoker! –Chef Philip

Grilled Pork with Savory, Cardamom & Cumin

Gluten-Free, Dairy-Free

Makes 8–10 servings | 190 calories per serving

¼ cup olive oil

1–2 pork tenderloins

1–2 teaspoons sea salt

Savory, ground

Cardamom, ground

Cumin, ground

1. Put the oil on the bottom of a large dish and add the pork tenderloins.
2. With a fork, turn the pork so that it gets lightly coated with the oil; add the salt while turning.
3. Next, sprinkle the three spices liberally on the pork, on at least two sides.
4. Cover tightly with plastic wrap and refrigerate. This meat can stay in the refrigerator for up to 2 days.
5. Preheat the grill on high and when hot, sear the tenderloins for 3–5 minutes on each side.
6. Remove the pork from the grill, cover with foil, and let rest about 5 minutes.
7. Turn down the heat to medium. (If your grill has a temperature gauge, you sear at about 700°F and then cook over medium at 300–400°F.)
8. When the grill is ready, put the pork back on the grill for 20–30 minutes, turning once or twice.
9. When done, place on a cutting board for a few minutes before cutting into ½-inch slices.

Notes: This combination of spices is great with pork, and this dish is just as good with thick, on-the-bone pork chops as it is with pork tenderloins. In any case, try to get good-quality, lean pork. • This process—searing on high heat (about 700 °F) on all sides first, and then cooking the meat through at a lower temperature (300–400°F)—works for almost every meat that can be grilled. • Get to know your grill: If it is very slow cooling down after the searing stage, actually take the meat off and let it sit for 5 minutes covered with foil until the grill temperature is medium-hot. • By the way, this recipe is designed for a gas grill; it can be cooked on a regular charcoal grill, but it takes more skill not to burn the meat. • This recipe is intended for cooking on an outdoor grill, but it can be cooked inside on the stove and in the oven: Preheat the oven to 400°F, then sear the pork on the stovetop in a large frying pan to brown on all sides. (To do this on the stovetop, you may have to cut the pork into smaller pieces.) Then, bake in the oven for 15–20 minutes. • This dish goes well with grilled corn on the cob, eggplant, asparagus, and/or baked potatoes. –Dr. Jamie

Pumpkin Gnocchi with Pistachio Sauce

Vegan, Dairy-Free
Makes 4 servings | 380 calories per serving

Gnocchi

1 cup roasted pumpkin purée (page 222)

1 teaspoon sea salt

¼ teaspoon ground nutmeg

1 cup semolina flour[NGF]

Sauce

1 cup raw pistachios[PT]

1 teaspoon sea salt

2 cups soymilk

20 fresh sage leaves (preferably with stems attached)

½ teaspoon freshly grated nutmeg

Directions for the gnocchi

1. Combine the pumpkin with the salt and nutmeg and mix well. Slowly incor-porate the flour until you have a dough. The less flour you add, the lighter the gnocchi will be.
2. Let the dough rest, covered or wrapped, for a half hour.
3. Divide the dough into 4 equal-size portions.
4. Roll out each portion into 1-inch-diameter logs of dough, flouring lightly as needed.
5. Cut the logs into ¾-inch-long pieces to create the gnocchi.
6. Drop the gnocchi in boiling water. When they float, they are finished. Remove from the water, drain, and sauce immediately. Do NOT make in advance; make them as you are ready to serve them.

Directions for the sauce

1. In a cast-iron skillet over medium-low heat, toast the pistachios, stirring constantly until they smell aromatic. Remove from the heat and place in a blender with the salt and soymilk. Blend until smooth.
2. Transfer the pistachio purée into a saucepan and place over low heat.
3. Add the sage leaves and, stirring regularly, bring to a simmer. Cook, stirring, until the sauce thickens slightly.
4. Add the nutmeg, remove the sage leaves, and serve the sauce with the gnocchi.

Notes: A wonderful autumn dish from Italy! • Usually the sauce is made with walnuts, but pistachios or pine nuts can make a very nice substitute that is reflux-friendly. • As a variation, you can replace the sage with fresh rosemary or marjoram. The amount of flour needed for the gnocchi will vary depending on the moisture of the roasted pumpkin, the humidity of the air, and the temperature of the room. –Chef Philip

Turkey Burger Salad with Black Olives & Avocado

Gluten-Free, Dairy-Free
Makes 4 servings | 275 calories per serving

1 pound ground turkey (preferably 93% lean/7% fat, as 99% lean can be too dry), formed into 4 patties

½ teaspoon sea salt

2 heads romaine lettuce, washed and cut or torn into 2- to 3-inch pieces

1 medium-size can of small, pitted black olives[PT]

2 tablespoons extra-virgin olive oil

1 teaspoon balsamic vinegar [PT, MMGF]

1 avocado, peeled and sliced

1. Season the turkey patties with the salt and cook on the grill or on the stovetop in a covered frying pan, over medium to medium-high heat for 4–5 minutes per side.
2. After cooking, put the burgers aside until cool enough to break into bite-size pieces.
3. Place the lettuce, olives, oil, and vinegar in a large salad bowl and toss.
4. Finally, add the burger pieces and avocado slices on top.

Notes: Turkey burgers are a good source of protein, but for people who are gluten-free, bread doesn't work. • The burgers go nicely with the vinaigrette and the black olives. • The avocado gives a nice contrasting texture and flavor. • Obviously this salad can be enhanced any number of ways, but I sometimes like to add sautéed mushrooms; if I do, I leave off the avocado. • Another nice variation is to add cucumber and red pepper (if not triggers). –Dr. Jamie

Gluten-Free Pasta with Shrimp & Zucchini

Gluten-Free, Dairy-Free, Detox-Friendly
Makes 6 servings | 460 calories per serving

1 pound gluten-free white-rice spaghetti

3–4 medium-size zucchinis, halved lengthwise and then sliced into ¼-inch half-moons

½ teaspoon sea salt

4 tablespoons olive oil

1½–2 pounds shrimp (fresh or frozen, uncooked or cooked), peeled and deveined

¾ cup chopped fresh basil leaves, stems removed

1. Get all of the ingredients ready at the start, because the sauce will take about the same time as the pasta to cook. If the shrimp are frozen, defrost them in cold water and then dry them.
2. Put a large pasta pot filled two-thirds with water over high heat.
3. When the water comes to a vigorous, rolling boil, put the pasta in.
4. Start the sauce when the pasta goes into the boiling water.
5. Salt the zucchini. In a large saucepan over high heat, place half of the olive oil and then add the zucchini. Brown the zucchini slices, turning them with a spatula; try not to "boil" them, which is why a big pan and high heat is best.
6. When the zucchini are almost done, add the shrimp. If they are raw, add more of the olive oil, if needed, then add the basil. Cook until heated through.
7. When the pasta is done, drain and serve in individual bowls.
8. Top with the shrimp and zucchini.

*Notes: This is a reflux-friendly, gluten-free spaghetti dish that is easy and fast. •
It is remarkable how good rice pasta is, and it reheats well also. • Don't worry
about how much olive oil you use, because it really does not cause reflux. (And,
by the way, if you regularly use butter, olive oil is always a great substitute; you
can use it on everything—pasta, meat, potatoes, fish, veggies, rice, etc.) • Think
about the endless variations of this dish: You can use other vegetables—carrots,
spinach, anything. And if you have leftover meat or fish, you can use that instead
of shrimp. I once made this with cod, snow peas, and cilantro. –Dr. Jamie*

Poached Arctic Char with Dill

Gluten-Free, Dairy-Free, Detox-Friendly
Makes 2–4 servings | 210 calories per serving

1 pound Arctic char, skin on

1–2 teaspoons olive oil

1 teaspoon sea salt

1 cup chicken or vegetable stock (page 217)

2 teaspoons minced fresh dill, stems removed

1. Cut the fish in half so that it will fit neatly in your pan, or you may cut it into individual servings.
2. Cover both sides of the fish lightly with the olive oil and then the salt.
3. Heat a shallow pan over medium-high heat, and then add the fish skin-side up.
4. Sauté for 2–3 minutes, until there is some sizzle.
5. Add the chicken stock and half of the dill.
6. When the stock is boiling lightly and steaming, cover the pan with a lid or foil. (If the steaming around the edges of the pan is excessive, lower the heat slightly.)
7. Cook for 12–18 minutes, until the fish skin peels off very easily; that's how you know it is done.
8. Plate and garnish with the rest of the fresh dill.

Notes: Store-bought vegetable stock usually contains onions, so if onion is a trigger for you, definitely use homemade. Or you may use chicken stock, store-bought or homemade; store-bought chicken stock is available without onions or sugar, for example. • We think that grilled or baked fish usually trumps poached fish, but this Arctic char recipe is a big exception. (Another exception is the Poached Halibut with Prosciutto recipe on page 177.) Arctic char is a delicious, light, flavorful, and delicate fish with exceptionally pleasing texture. • You may substitute any other fish-friendly spice for the dill if you prefer (like basil). • This Arctic char dish goes extremely well with the Rice with Cumin & Turmeric dish (page 151), as well as with sautéed or roasted vegetables such as eggplant, string beans, or asparagus. • This same dish can be made with salmon, as long as it is not too thick (less than 1½ inches thick). –Dr. Jamie

Steamed Sea Bass with Ginger & Soy

Gluten-Free, Dairy-Free
Makes 4 servings | 380 calories per serving

2 pounds sea bass fillet (or any flaky white fish)

2 teaspoons sea salt

1-inch piece fresh ginger, peeled and julienned

1 ½ tablespoons rice wine^{PT} (or any cooking wine)

2 tablespoons tamari (gluten-free soy sauce)

4 teaspoons toasted sesame oil^{PT} (optional)

1 tablespoon olive oil

½ cup fresh cilantro sprigs

1. Salt both sides of the fillet.
2. Scatter ginger over top of the fish.
3. Drizzle the rice wine over the fish and place on a heat-proof dish for steaming. Place in a steamer and cover. Steam for 15 minutes. Pour the water out of the dish.
4. Drizzle the tamari over the fish.
5. Heat the toasted sesame oil and olive oil in a pan over medium-high heat until they begin to smoke.
6. Carefully pour the oil on top of the fish.
7. Garnish with cilantro and serve immediately.

Notes: A variation of this aromatic sea bass dish is made all over China. • A firm white-fleshed fish, such as cod or halibut, may be substituted for the sea bass. • Sesame oil may be a trigger for some people. • Alternatively, this dish can be made by poaching the fish in ½ cup chicken or vegetable stock in a pan on the stovetop. –Sonia

Stir-Fried Rice Noodles with Vegetables

Vegan, Gluten-Free, Dairy-Free, Detox-Friendly
Makes 4 servings | 300 calories per serving

½ pound dried rice noodles

2 tablespoons olive oil

2 tablespoons minced fresh ginger

4 shiitake mushrooms, thinly sliced

1 carrot, julienned

1 cup sliced choy sum or bok choy,
1-inch slivers

½ cup chopped fresh basil

2 tablespoons tamari (gluten-free soy
sauce)

2 teaspoons palm sugar

1 tablespoon shaoshing wine [PT, MMGF]
or dry sherry[PT] (optional; see note)

⅓ cup seaweed-mushroom or vegetable
stock (pages 217–218)

1. Pour boiling water over the rice noodles in a bowl. Let soak for 2–5 minutes, or until the noodles are soft; do NOT oversoak. Drain, rinse under cold water, and set aside.
2. In a hot wok or skillet over medium-high heat, add the oil and ginger and stir-fry for 1 minute.
3. Add the shiitake, carrots, choy sum, and basil. Continue stir-frying for 3 minutes.
4. Add the rest of the ingredients and bring to a boil, stirring constantly.
5. Add the drained rice noodles and mix gently. Serve very hot.

Notes: Rice noodles have a wonderful texture and are gluten-free; they have been made in China and Southeast Asia for millennia. • This dish is known as Chow Fun in China and Pad Kee Mao in Thailand. • We decided to rate this recipe as detox-friendly, because the amount of wine is so small (and it can be omitted). —Chef Philip

Clams with Basil & Ginger

Gluten-Free, Dairy-Free, Detox-Friendly
Makes 4 servings | 170 calories per serving

1 tablespoon olive oil

2 cloves garlic[PT] (optional; see note)

1-inch piece fresh ginger, peeled and julienned

1 pound clams, cleaned

1 tablespoon rice wine[PT] (optional; see note)

2 tablespoons tamari (gluten-free soy sauce)

1 teaspoon sugar

2 tablespoons water

Pinch of salt to taste

½ cup basil leaves

1. Heat the oil in a pan over medium-high heat, then add the garlic and ginger and stir-fry until fragrant, 1 minute. Remove and discard the garlic cloves.
2. Add the clams and stir-fry over high heat until the shells start to open.
3. Add the rice wine, tamari, sugar, and water. Stir-fry until the sauce is almost dry, then season to taste with salt. Discard any clams that haven't opened.
4. Add the basil and serve.

Notes: If the rice wine and garlic are omitted, this dish is detox-friendly • This healthy and flavorful dish is very quick to make. • The fragrant basil makes a huge difference. • I prefer to use Chinese basil or Thai basil, but if you cannot find them in your local Asian market, you can substitute Italian basil. • Chinese basil is similar to Thai basil but is much sweeter. —Sonia

Stir-Fried Shrimp & Peas

Gluten-Free, Dairy-Free, Detox-Friendly
Makes 4 servings | 320 calories per serving

1¼ teaspoons salt

2 tablespoons cornstarch[MMGF]

1 tablespoon rice wine[PT] (optional; see note)

1 pound uncooked shrimp, peeled and deveined

¼ cup olive oil

6 ounces frozen corn

6 ounces frozen peas

1. Combine 1 teaspoon of the salt with the cornstarch and rice wine in a bowl. Add the shrimp and marinate for 10 minutes.
2. Heat the olive oil in a pan over medium-high and sauté the shrimp until opaque.
3. Stir in the corn and peas and cook until heated through.
4. Season with ¼ teaspoon salt (or to taste) and serve.

Notes: If the rice wine is omitted, this dish is detox-friendly. • An extremely quick and easy dish to make after a long day. • Stir-frying is a traditional Asian cooking technique that uses very little oil in a hot wok to cook the food while quickly stirring. • This type of cooking seals in the freshness while retaining the vibrant colors of the food. • Because it only takes a few minutes to cook, it is best to have all the ingredients ready before firing up the wok. —Sonia

Braised Pork with Carrots & Daikon

Gluten-Free, Dairy-Free
Makes 8 servings | 400 calories per serving

1 tablespoon olive oil

5 (⅛-inch-thick) slices peeled fresh ginger

2 pounds pork loin, cut into 1½-inch pieces

1 cup shaoshing wine ᴾᵀ, ᴹᴹᴳᶠ or dry sherryᴾᵀ

2½ tablespoons tamari (gluten-free soy sauce)

3 star anise

8 cloves

1 teaspoon honey

5 cups water

½ large daikon radish, cut into 1½-inch pieces (about 2 cups; if unavailable, substitute turnips)

½ large carrot, cut into 1½-inch pieces

Handful of fresh cilantro, chopped

1. Heat the oil in a Dutch oven or a large pan over medium-high heat. Add the ginger and sauté for 1 minute, or until fragrant.
2. Add the pork and sauté until browned on all sides.
3. Add the wine, tamari, star anise, cloves, honey, and water. Cover and cook until the pork is tender, adding more water if needed.
4. Add the daikon and carrots and cook uncovered until the liquid is reduced by half and the veggies are cooked through. Remove the star anise and cloves and discard.
5. Sprinkle with cilantro and serve hot.

Notes: This is a super easy and tasty comfort food dish that brings fond memories of father and daughter time. • As a treat, my dad would take me to the local bookstore, where I could buy whatever book I fancied, followed by a big bowl of irresistibly yummy braised beef with turnips over rice from the local market. • Here, I've replaced the beef shin that the traditional dish calls for with lean pork loin. –Sonia

Linguine with Mussels & Arugula

Dairy-Free, Detox-Friendly
Makes 4 servings | 480 calories per serving

¼ cup olive oil

3 large cloves garlic^{PT} (optional; see note)

24 mussels, scrubbed and debearded

2 cups vegetable stock (page 217)

½ pound linguine,^{NGF} cooked

2 cups (packed) baby arugula

Salt to taste

1. Heat the oil in a large sauté pan over medium-high heat.

2. Sauté the garlic cloves for 2 minutes, then remove and discard the cloves.

3. Add the mussels and vegetable stock, cover, and cook for 5–8 minutes, until the mussels open up. Discard any mussels that haven't opened.

4. Add the linguine and arugula and stir together.

5. Season with salt to taste and serve hot.

Notes: If the garlic is omitted, this dish is detox-friendly. • This is a quick and easy summer recipe. • If you are gluten-free, you can substitute rice noodle linguine. –Sonia

HORS D'OEUVRES & SNACKS

Skillet Cornbread

Vegan, Dairy-Free, Detox-Friendly
Makes 4 servings | 175 calories per serving

Grapeseed oil, for coating skillet

1 cup yellow cornmeal[MMGF]

1 cup white flour[NGF]

1 tablespoon baking powder[MMGF]

½ teaspoon sea salt

1¼ cups soymilk

3 tablespoons olive oil

2 tablespoons maple syrup

1. Coat a 9-inch cast-iron skillet in grapeseed oil, then preheat the skillet in a 425°F oven for a half hour.
2. Whisk together the dry ingredients in a bowl and set aside.
3. Put the soymilk, olive oil, and maple syrup in a blender and blend until smooth.
4. Add the wet ingredients to the dry. Mix lightly to combine, but do not over-mix!
5. Remove the skillet from the oven (leave the oven on) and carefully coat it in grapeseed oil.
6. Pour the batter into the well-oiled, HOT cast-iron pan. Cook on the stovetop a few minutes over medium-low heat, until bubbles start to appear on the surface.
7. Then bake for 30 minutes, or until a toothpick inserted in the center comes out clean.

Notes: A cast-iron skillet produces the best texture, but if you do not have one, you can use a 9 x 13-inch glass baking dish. The texture will be very different, but the flavor will remain the same. (The skillet makes it crunchy.) • Option 1 (not for detox diet): add 1 red apple, peeled, cored, and grated, to the wet mix. Option 2: sauté the kernels from 1 ear of corn and/or 1 chopped red pepper (not for detox diet) in 1 tablespoon olive oil for 3 minutes. Add this to the batter and then cook as directed above. —Chef Philip

Pearl Balls

Gluten-Free, Dairy-Free
Makes 8 servings | 200 calories per serving

1 cup short-grain Asian rice (sticky rice)

4 dried shiitake mushrooms

1½ pounds ground chicken or turkey

½ pound ground shrimp

2 teaspoons finely grated fresh ginger

3 teaspoons tamari (gluten-free soy sauce)

2 teaspoons sake[PT]

1 teaspoon toasted sesame oil[PT]

1 teaspoon honey

1 teaspoon salt

1 tablespoon cornstarch[MMGF]

3 large cabbage leaves

1. Soak the rice in enough water to cover for 4 hours. Drain and pat dry. Set aside.
2. In warm water, soak the mushrooms until soft. Rinse the mushrooms and pat dry. Remove the stems and finely chop the caps.
3. Combine the mushrooms with the remaining ingredients (except the rice and cabbage leaves) in a bowl and mix until well blended. Form the mixture into balls 1 inch in diameter.
4. Coat each ball completely with rice.
5. Line a steamer with the cabbage leaves and set the pearl balls on top. Steam the pearl balls in a pan or wok for 30 minutes. Serve hot.

Notes: This traditional steamed Asian dish got its name because the rice looks like little pearls studded over the juicy chicken balls. • These make a fabulous appetizer for any dinner party, as they present exquisitely. –Sonia

Marbled Tea Eggs

Vegetarian, Gluten-Free, Dairy-Free
Makes 6 servings | 70 calories per serving

6 eggs, hard-boiled

¾ cup tamari (gluten-free soy sauce)

1 cup water

½-inch piece fresh ginger, sliced

2 black tea[PT] bags (optional)

½ teaspoon Chinese spice blend (page 220)

1. Crack the hard-boiled eggs well but do not peel. This will give the eggs a mottled look.
2. Add the eggs to a pot with the tamari, water, ginger, black tea bags, and Chinese spice blend. Make sure that the liquid completely covers the eggs and add more water if needed.
3. Simmer over low heat for 25 minutes, then let the eggs steep for 30 minutes. Remove from the liquid and let cool.
4. When cool, peel the eggs and slice into wedges to serve.

Notes: This famous Chinese street food was one of my favorite snacks growing up. • The staining and cracking process creates a beautiful marbled effect. • Serve them as a snack or a whimsical addition to breakfast or brunch. • Black tea may be a trigger food for some people and may be omitted. —Sonia

Royal Caviar Egg Treat

Gluten-Free, Dairy-Free
Makes 1 serving | 170 calories per serving

3 jumbo hard-boiled eggs
1 small jar salmon roe (caviar)

1. Peel the eggs and slice them in half crosswise. Scoop out the yolks.
2. Line up the six egg halves, leaning them against each other so they stand up. (Using a sharp knife, you can cut the tip off the pointy end so that it stands up more easily.)
3. Finely chop one of the yolks and with the knife place some yolk in each egg half.
4. Top each mound of yolk liberally with caviar.

Notes: You don't have to use jumbo eggs, but that is all I use because the yolk is generally the same in different-size eggs, so the jumbos just have more egg white. • *For easy-to-peel hard-boiled eggs, don't use recently bought eggs; eggs that are at least a week old simply peel better.* • *Also, after they are boiled, cool them quickly and get them in the refrigerator.* • *Relatively inexpensive salmon roe is great; don't buy expensive caviar for this snack.* • *This might be a treat at work and can be served to company as an hors d'oeuvre.* • *If you are serving caviar eggs to company, cut the pointy bottoms square so that they stand up on a plate.* • *Also, place a cocktail napkin or a small doily on each plate to keep the eggs from sliding around.* • *These look and taste special—hence "Royal." –Dr. Jamie*

Popcorn with Rosemary & Salt

Vegan, Gluten-Free, Dairy-Free, Detox-Friendly

Makes 4 servings | 100 calories per serving

2 tablespoons olive oil

½ cup popping corn

1 teaspoon sea salt

2 teaspoons nutritional yeast

1/3 teaspoon powdered rosemary

1. In a hot pot over medium heat, add the olive oil and popping corn. Cover tightly. Shake the pot until you hear the corn start to pop and then stop popping.
2. Remove from the heat and add the rest of the ingredients.
3. Turn on a movie and enjoy the popcorn.

Notes: Nutritional yeast is different from baking yeast and is easy to find in bulk sections of grocery stores. • It is gluten-free, and it adds a "cheesy" flavor to a dish.• It also provides a lot of B vitamins. –Chef Philip

Beet Nut Pâté

Vegan, Gluten-Free, Dairy-Free

Makes 4 servings | 345 calories per serving

½ cup raw pine nuts

½ cup raw sunflower seeds

½ cup raw pistachios^PT

½ cup raw pumpkin seeds

1 tablespoon tamari (gluten-free soy sauce)

¾ cup grated raw purple beets

½ red bell pepper^PT

½ small carrot

2-inch piece daikon radish

20 fresh basil leaves

Salt to taste (optional)

1. Place all of the ingredients except the salt in a food processor and purée until smooth. Add a little bit of water if needed.
2. Season with salt if desired.

Notes: This is a wonderful spread for fresh bread or a great accompaniment to a buffet, providing a bright purple color and complex flavors. –Chef Philip

Garbanzo (Socca) Crepes with Smoked Eggplant Spread & Vegetables

Vegan, Gluten-Free, Dairy-Free

Makes 4 servings | 175 calories per serving

Crepes

2 cups garbanzo bean flour

2 cups water

2 tablespoons olive oil

2 teaspoons sea salt

1 tablespoon dried sage

1 tablespoon dried rosemary

Vegetables

1 tablespoon olive oil

1 carrot, julienned

10 snow peas, julienned

10 medium stalks asparagus, julienned

½ teaspoon sea salt

2 tablespoons raw pine nuts

2 teaspoons balsamic vinegar PT, MMGF

Spread

2 large whole eggplants, cap and stem intact

1 teaspoon grapeseed oil

½ teaspoon sea salt

Apple wood or alder wood, for smoking

1 teaspoon salt

1 teaspoon ground cumin

1 teaspoon sweet paprikaPT

1 whole raw tomatoPT

Directions for the crepes

1. In a bowl, whisk together all of the crepe ingredients. Cover and let rest for 2 hours.
2. Over medium heat, warm up a cast-iron pan or crepe pan for 10 minutes.
3. Coat the pan with olive oil.
4. Whisk the crepe batter well and then ladle about ½ cup of the mixture into the center of the pan, making a circle extending outward until the batter thinly coats the pan by using the ladle or swirling the pan.
5. Cook over medium heat until it starts to bubble. Flip only once and cook on the other side about 1 minute.
6. Remove from the pan. Best served hot and crisp!

Notes: This is best cooked in a cast-iron or crepe pan. If not available, it can be baked in a baking dish. If baking, keep the batter thin (1/8-inch maximum thickness in pan) for best texture and flavor.

Directions for the vegetables

1. In a hot skillet over medium heat, add the olive oil.
2. Add the carrot, snow peas, and asparagus and sauté for 2 minutes.
3. Add the sea salt and pine nuts and sauté for 2 more minutes.
4. Add the balsamic vinegar and mix well.
5. Reserve hot, warm, or at room temperature.

Notes: Always use what is in season! In the spring, I like to use asparagus, snow peas, and carrots. In the fall and winter, replace the asparagus with thinly julienned kabocha squash or cubes of butternut squash. In the summer, I replace the asparagus with the kernels from 2 ears of corn for great texture!

Directions for the spread

1. Rub a little grapeseed oil and ½ teaspoon sea salt on the eggplants.
2. Smoke the eggplants, using apple wood or alder wood or a combination, until the eggplants totally collapse.
3. Remove and discard the charred skin.
4. Place the flesh of the eggplants with the rest of the ingredients in a food processor and purée until smooth.

Notes: Smoking takes eggplants to a whole new level! Smoking provides a primal flavor, perhaps the second flavor humans experienced after raw. I never miss any meat flavors, but once I started smoking tempeh, tofu, and vegetables, I realized how much I had missed smoked flavors! Outdoor grills are ideal for smoking foods. Stovetop smokers are available for inside the home, or you can easily rig up a smoker using a wok, chopsticks, and a wok lid.

Directions for serving

1. Smear the smoked eggplant spread on a crepe and top with the sautéed vegetable mixture. Cut into 4–8 sections like a pizza.

(continued on next page)

Notes: Socca is a flat bread or crepe made from garbanzo beans from southern France, influenced and developed by Arab immigrants. • This is one of the most popular finger foods on my catering menu. • We serve this at practically every catering event, varying the toppings based on the season. • Socca is a wonderful fancy appetizer for a party. • Although it requires several steps, each step is fairly easy, and the results are colorful and flavorful, and they will wow your guests. –Chef Philip

Turkey Lettuce Cups with Pine Nuts

Dairy-Free
Makes 8 servings | 200 calories per serving

2 teaspoons olive oil

1-inch piece peeled fresh ginger, diced

1 pound ground turkey

2 tablespoons oyster sauce[NGF, PT]

2 tablespoons tamari (gluten-free soy sauce)

¼ cup finely sliced green beans

¾ cup raw pine nuts

Salt to taste

8 iceberg lettuce leaves

¼ cup shredded carrots

1. Heat the oil in a large sauté pan over medium-high heat, then add the ginger and cook until fragrant.
2. Add the ground turkey and sauté until the turkey is browned.
3. Add the oyster sauce, tamari, green beans, pine nuts, and salt to taste. Cook, stirring, for 2 minutes.
4. Divide the mixture between the lettuce leaves, top with the shredded carrots, and roll up as best as you can.

Note: These wraps are delicious and bursting with flavor. • The clean crispness of the lettuce and the crunch of pine nuts play well with the saltiness of the turkey mixture. • Can be made into beautifully tantalizing bite-size appetizers by trimming the lettuce to the desired size, or serve family-style and let everyone make their own. –Sonia

DESSERTS

Kick-Ass Carrot Cookies

Vegan, Dairy-Free
Makes 3 dozen cookies | 65 calories per cookie

1 cup rolled oats^{MMGF}

1 cup white flour^{NGF}

1 teaspoon ground cinnamon

1 teaspoon baking powder^{MMGF}

½ teaspoon baking soda^{MMGF}

¼ teaspoon salt

½ cup maple syrup

½ cup grapeseed oil

1 cup grated carrot

½ cup dried cherries^{PT} (see note)

1. Preheat the oven to 375°F.
2. In one bowl, combine the oats, flour, cinnamon, baking powder, baking soda, and salt.
3. In a separate bowl, whisk together the syrup and oil.
4. Add the carrots and dried cherries to the wet mixture and mix well.
5. Pour the wet mixture over the dry mixture and gently combine. Do NOT over-mix, or the cookies will be rubbery.
6. Drop 1-teaspoon portions of the mixture on a grapeseed-oiled baking sheet, 2 inches apart. (These cookies only bake well if they are small.)
7. Bake for 10 minutes. Be careful not to overcook, as they burn easily.

Notes: For the picky eaters in your home, sneak a little carrot into their diet with this amazing cookie recipe. • For a fun variation, dried cherries can be replaced by currants, raisins, dried blueberries, or dried cranberries, or a combination. – Chef Philip

Seared Watermelon with Feta & Prosciutto

Gluten-Free
Makes 2 servings | 75 calories per serving

8 (½-inch by ½-inch by 2–3-inch-long) rectangular solids (like square logs),
  cut from the heart of half a watermelon, avoiding seeds
4 thin slices prosciutto[PT]
2 teaspoons crumbled feta cheese

1. Place a medium-size frying pan over high heat.
2. When the pan is quite hot, spray it with nonstick cooking spray and place four of the watermelon logs in the frying pan.
3. Turn the logs to sear each of the four sides. If the pan is hot enough, it is about 30 seconds per side. (You want them just to sear a bit, no more.)
4. When the first four watermelon logs have a smidge of black on all sides, remove from the heat and set aside.
5. Repeat the same procedure with the remaining four watermelon logs.
6. To plate, neatly place two pieces of prosciutto on each 8-inch plate and then stack four watermelon logs (two on top of two) per serving on the prosciutto.
7. Garnish each watermelon tower with a teaspoon of feta.

Notes: This is a really fun dish to make with your dinner company watching you. Everyone always seems surprised that you can cook watermelon. • The caramelized taste of the watermelon is unique, and the combination of all the ingredients is light but savory. • One could use crumbled tofu or sprinkle nutritional yeast instead of the feta if you are dairy-free. –Dr. Jamie

Poached Pears with Tea & Vanilla

Vegan, Gluten-Free, Dairy-Free
Makes 4 servings | 163 calories per serving

1 quart water

2 vanilla beans, split in half

3 cardamom pods

1 cinnamon stick

2 cloves

½ cup maple syrup

2 tablespoons jasmine tea leaves,[PT] or
4 jasmine tea bags[PT] (oolong[PT] can be
substituted)

2 large pears,[PT] halved and cored

1. Bring the water to a boil.
2. Add the vanilla, cardamom, cinnamon, cloves, syrup, and tea.
3. Cover, remove from the heat, and let sit for 10 minutes. Remove the tea
   (if you have not used tea bags, strain to remove the loose tea leaves).
4. Bring back to a simmer.
5. Add the pears, cover, and cook over low heat for 20 minutes.

*Notes: The fruit absorbs liquid as it is being poached and becomes very tender. •
Poaching is a great way to add lots of flavor to fruit, and a good poaching liquid
is vital, as the fruit will take on its flavor. • Wonderful by itself, but even better
served with ice cream or sorbet. —Chef Philip*

Banana Pistachio Ice Cream

Vegan, Gluten-Free, Dairy-Free
Makes 8 servings | 150 calories per serving

½ cup raw pistachios[PT]

2 cups water

½ cup maple syrup

4 ripe bananas

½ teaspoon ground cinnamon

1. Place all of the ingredients in a blender and purée until totally smooth.
2. Transfer the purée to an ice cream maker and churn until frozen according to the manufacturer's instructions.

Notes: Going vegan became easy when I learned how to make ice creams out of nuts. • As a vegan chef, I find cashews to be a solution for many culinary needs. • Raw cashews provide a great deal of fat yet very little flavor, thus making them ideal for sauces and ice creams and many other applications. • However, for reflux diets, cashews may be a trigger, so we have replaced them with pistachios in this recipe. As nuts go, pistachios are an uncommon reflux trigger, so this ice cream may be suitable for most people on the detox diet—I consider this only a minor cheat. • This handcrafted vegan ice cream is a signature of my underground restaurant and catering menus, often surprising and even shocking many of the omnivore diners. —Chef Philip

Caramelized Bananas

Vegan, Gluten-Free, Dairy-Free, Detox-Friendly
Makes 4 servings | 110 calories per serving

¼ cup palm sugar
¼ cup water
2 bananas, halved lengthwise

1. In a small frying pan over medium-low heat, combine the sugar and water, stirring until the sugar dissolves.
2. Add the bananas, cook for 5 minutes, and then turn over and cook another 5 minutes.

Notes: Everyone deserves a treat, and there's certainly something that conquers images of the extravagant and the luxurious with this dish. • I'm sure Elvis would have enjoyed this as a snack! It goes particularly well on pancakes or crepes. • For extra flavor, add a split vanilla bean or a cinnamon stick to the sugar water mixture as the sugar dissolves. –Chef Philip

Watermelon Sorbet

Vegan, Gluten-Free, Dairy-Free, Detox-Friendly
Makes 4 servings | 15 calories per serving

4 cups watermelon purée
1 tablespoon lemon zest

1. Combine the watermelon purée and lemon zest and freeze in an ice cream maker according to the manufacturer's instructions.

Notes: It will be hard to find something more refreshing and quenching in the summer than this insanely simple-to-create dish. • Purée the watermelon in a high-speed blender. • Lemon zest is fine for refluxers; it's the juice and fruit that cause problems, not the peel. –Chef Philip

Ginger-Carrot Ice Pop

Vegan, Gluten-Free, Dairy-Free, Detox-Friendly
Makes 2 servings | 160 calories per serving

2 tablespoons agave

2 cups fresh carrot juice

2 teaspoons fresh ginger juice

1. Mix all of the ingredients together and pour into an ice pop mold. Insert sticks and freeze until set.

Notes: Late one evening, while chatting with my dear friend Chris about parenting, he mentioned a healthy and cheap alternative to buying store-bought ice pops for his two little boys. • I was intrigued, and inspired by the image of their little hands reaching into the freezer for a bright, multicolored selection of treats—so healthy that they can be enjoyed after breakfast. I decided to make them for my children. Instant hit! • You really need a juicer for this recipe; the juices should be fresh. • If you want to make more, you can obviously double or triple this recipe. –Sonia

Cucumber Cooler

Vegan, Gluten-Free, Dairy-Free, Detox-Friendly
Makes 4 servings | 20 calories per serving

2 cucumbers (preferably Japanese or Persian), peeled

4 quarts water

1. Purée the cucumbers in a blender with a little of the water until smooth.
2. Combine the purée with the rest of the water.
3. Pour over ice and serve.

Notes: A simple and very refreshing summertime drink! • Add rosemary sprigs or lime zest for some playful options. –Chef Philip

Cucumber Sorbet

Vegan, Gluten-Free, Dairy-Free, Detox-Friendly
Makes 4 servings | 50 calories per serving

2 pounds cucumbers (preferably Japanese or Persian), peeled

1 cup water

1 teaspoon lemon zest

2 tablespoons maple syrup (optional; this works without any sweetener)

1. Place all of the ingredients in a blender and purée until smooth.
2. Transfer purée to an ice cream maker and churn until frozen according to manufacturer's instructions.

Notes: This is a great summer refresher on a sweltering summer evening, as the cucumbers have an immediate cooling effect on the body. • The clean, refreshing taste of the sorbet also makes a great palate refresher. • For a fun serving idea, scoop the sorbet into hollowed-out lime halves. –Chef Philip

Natural Fruit Mold

Vegan, Gluten-Free, Dairy-Free
Makes 4 servings | 70 calories per serving

2 cups water
1 cup fresh blueberry juice[PT]
2 teaspoons kanten (agar) powder
Fresh seasonal fruit, sliced
Seasonal berries[PT]

1. In a saucepan, heat up the water and juice, then add the kanten powder and stir constantly with a whisk to dissolve.
2. Bring the mixture to a boil, lower the heat, and cook, stirring constantly, for 3 minutes.
3. Pour the kanten mixture into a 9 x 13-inch glass baking dish.
4. Decorate with fresh fruit slices and berries.
5. Let set for 2 hours, then chill before serving.

Notes: This is a very refreshing summer dish from Japan, and it is quite simple and inexpensive to prepare. • Kanten has an immediate cooling effect on the body and is also very good for digestion. • Multiple layers of kanten can be prepared for a very beautiful plate. After you prepare one layer, let it fully set and then prepare the second layer. • When doing this, use different juices with different colors so that each layer has a different color. –Chef Philip

Shaved Fruit Ice

Vegetarian, Gluten-Free, Dairy-Free
Makes 4 servings | 120 calories per serving

4 cups crushed ice

4 tablespoons honey

4 tablespoons vanilla almond milk

2 cups diced seasonal fruits

1. Divide the crushed ice equally into four serving cups.

2. Drizzle 1 tablespoon honey and 1 tablespoon almond milk over each ice cup.

3. Top each with ½ cup diced fruits.

Notes: This traditional Taiwanese summer treat is traditionally topped with sweetened beans, taro root, and jellies and is drizzled with sugar syrup and condensed milk. • My favorite variation as a child was one made with sweet preserved plums, as the acidity balanced out the sweetness of the traditional treat. • Before I immigrated to the U.S., shaved ice using "milk ice" had just started to become popular in Taiwan. Milk ice makes a more finely shaved, cold fluffy goodness that looks like a cloud covered in jewels (fruits). • This healthier version replaces the traditional condensed milk and sugar syrup with vanilla almond milk and a bit of honey, but still offers a satisfying, cool, sweet reward on a hot day. –Sonia

KITCHEN STAPLES

Vegetable Stock

Vegan, Gluten-Free, Dairy-Free, Detox-Friendly

3 dried shiitake mushrooms

1 carrot, peeled and coarsely chopped

1 stalk celery, coarsely chopped

1 potato, peeled and coarsely chopped

¼ cup parsley stems

2–3 (6-inch) square pieces kombu
  (a type of Japanese seaweed; optional)

1 teaspoon sea salt

2 quarts water

1. In a small stockpot, add the mushrooms, carrot, celery, potato, parsley stems, kombu, salt, and water.
2. Bring to a boil, cover, lower the heat, and let simmer for 30 minutes.
3. Simmer longer for a deeper flavor.

Chicken Stock

Gluten-Free, Dairy-Free, Detox-Friendly

5 quarts cold water

4 ½–5-pound chicken, cut into 8 pieces, excess skin and fat removed

1 tablespoon salt

1-pound yam, peeled, halved crosswise

¾ pound carrots, peeled, thickly sliced

½ pound parsnips, peeled, thickly sliced

4 large stalks celery, cut into 2-inch pieces

12 large fresh dill sprigs

12 large fresh parsley sprigs

Lemon zest of 1 lemon

1. Bring the water to a boil in a stockpot.
2. Add the chicken and return to a boil, skimming any impurities, for 15 minutes. Add the yam, carrots, parsnips, and celery. Reduce the heat to medium-low and gently simmer for 1 ½ hours.
3. Add the dill, parsley, and lemon zest and simmer for 3 minutes.
4. Remove from the heat and let stand for an hour, then strain. Store stock in the refrigerator for up to 2 days or freeze for up to 1 month.

Seaweed-Mushroom Stock (kombu dashi)

Vegan, Gluten-Free, Dairy-Free, Detox-Friendly

A very easy and flavorful stock that can be used in almost all savory dishes requiring stock. This is the base stock for my other stocks. By adding more ingredients (vegetables, vegetable parts, spices, herbs), we can produce very different-flavored stocks.

Seaweed-mushroom stock uses two inexpensive Japanese ingredients, both easy to find at Japanese or Asian markets and at many grocery stores. These days, we can easily find any ingredient online.

3 dried shiitake mushrooms
2–3 6-inch square pieces kombu (a type of Japanese seaweed)
1 teaspoon sea salt
2 quarts water

1. In a small stockpot, add the mushrooms, kombu, and water.
2. Bring to a boil, cover, lower the heat, and let simmer for 30 minutes.
3. Simmer longer for a deeper flavor.

Once you have seaweed-mushroom stock, you can make Miso Soup (page 109) in a couple of minutes.

Notes: Kombu is a seaweed (variety of kelp), and there are many varieties found off the coasts of Japan and Northern California. Easily found in Japanese markets or online, "dashi kombu" refers to kombu made for stocks and is worth seeking out and adding to your pantry. Kombu provides a tremendous amount of flavor and minerals that you may recognize from Japanese and Korean restaurants, as it is widely used in many stocks and dishes. Kombu, like all traditional Japanese ingredients, is widely known for its healing attributes, aiding in digesting plant proteins. –Chef Philip

Balsamic Vinegar & Oil Dressing

Vegan, Gluten-Free, Dairy-Free

2 tablespoons balsamic vinegar ^{PT, MMGF}

2 tablespoons olive oil

¼ teaspoon dried thyme

¼ teaspoon dried marjoram or oregano

½ teaspoon mustard powder

¼ teaspoon sea salt

1. Whisk all of the ingredients together in a bowl. Store covered in the refrigerator for up to 2 weeks.

Garlic-Oil Dressing

Vegan, Gluten-Free, Dairy-Free

2 tablespoons garlic-infused olive oil^{PT} (page 220)

1 teaspoon rice vinegar ^{PT, MMGF}

½ teaspoon sea salt

1. Whisk all of the ingredients together in a bowl. Store covered in the refrigerator for up to 2 weeks.

Sesame Dressing

Vegan, Gluten-Free, Dairy-Free

¼ cup toasted sesame seeds^{PT}

1 tablespoon seaweed-mushroom stock (page 218)

1 ½ tablespoons tamari (gluten-free soy sauce)

1 teaspoon sake^{PT}

1 tablespoon mirin^{PT}

1. Whisk all of the ingredients together in a bowl. Store covered in the refrigerator for up to 2 weeks.

Chinese Spice Blend

Vegan, Gluten-Free, Dairy-Free, Detox-Friendly

1 teaspoon ground cinnamon

½ teaspoon ground cloves

1 teaspoon fennel seeds, toasted and ground

1 teaspoon ground aniseed

½ teaspoon ground ginger

1. Mix all of the ingredients together in an airtight container and store for up to 1 month.

Garlic-Infused Olive Oil

Vegan, Gluten-Free, Dairy-Free

Handful of garlic cloves, peeled

Olive oil

1. Place several garlic cloves in olive oil (they should be covered) and let sit for a few days at room temperature.
2. Remove the cloves and discard.
3. Store the oil in the refrigerator and use within 2 weeks.

Notes: Use this whenever you want to add garlic flavor. Always add flavored oils at the end of a dish for best effect. Although many people who have acid reflux problems must avoid eating garlic, the infused oil often is not a trigger, thus providing the wonderful garlic flavor without the problem. –Chef Philip

Sauerkraut

Vegan, Gluten-Free, Dairy-Free, Detox-Friendly

5 pounds cabbage, shredded

3 tablespoons sea salt

1. Place the cabbage in a bowl and sprinkle with the salt.
2. Massage the salt into the cabbage for a few minutes, making sure that the cabbage is completely covered with the salt.
3. Pack the salted cabbage tightly into a crock.
4. Place a weight on the cabbage to keep it submerged in the liquid that it will expel as it ferments.
5. Cover loosely and let sit in a clean area for 1 month.
6. Skim off the top layer and enjoy the kraut.

Notes: Variations: add 2 tablespoons juniper berries, 1 tablespoon allspice berries, ½ cup chopped fresh dill, or 2 tablespoons caraway seeds to the kraut before packing into crock.• Sauerkraut, like all fermented foods, aids in digestion. For reflux diets, it should be used sparingly. —Chef Philip

How to Roast and Purée a Pumpkin

Vegan, Gluten-Free, Dairy-Free, Detox-Friendly

This is one of the most important fundamental recipes for the fall kitchen. Pumpkin is a wonderful, nutritious, and very flavorful American vegetable. There are a wide variety of pumpkins available in markets. The larger ones tend to be for carving and are good for seeds, but the meat tends to be tough, stringy, and not very flavorful. Small orange pumpkins, sometimes called "pie pumpkins" or "sugar pie pumpkins," are wonderful for most puréed-pumpkin needs, as are butternut squash and Cinderella pumpkins. Puréed pumpkin is so versatile and is used constantly in my kitchen during the fall and winter seasons for both savory and sweet dishes.

This takes a small amount of effort, but the results more than make up for it, especially in comparison to what one finds in a can on supermarket shelves.

1. Preheat the oven to 425°F.
2. Use a sugar pie pumpkin (small orange pumpkin).
3. Cut the pumpkin in half. Scoop out the seeds and membrane and save the seeds for roasting. The skin and gooey part can be used for a delicious pumpkin stock (page 114), so do not discard any part of the pumpkin!
4. Lightly salt the pumpkin, massaging the salt into the flesh.
5. Place the pumpkin in a roasting pan cut-side up, add ½ cup water to the pan, and cover tightly.
6. Roast for 45 minutes. Scoop the pumpkin flesh away from the skin and purée it in a food processor or mash with a potato masher or fork. Pies, sorbets, breads, soups, and so much more are now ready to be made with your pumpkin purée.

Notes: Pumpkin is one of my favorite vegetables, and I prepare dozens of pumpkin dishes, sweet and savory, every fall and winter. This is the first step for most of those dishes. —Chef Philip

Recipe Guide

V=Vegan, **Veg**=Vegetarian,
GF=Gluten-Free, **DF**=Dairy-Free, *=Detox-Friendly

Breakfast

Soups

Salads

Sides

Entrées

Snacks & Hors D'oeuvres

Desserts

Kitchen Staples

Ingredient List and the Recipes that Use Them

NGF Not gluten-free.

MMGF May or may not be gluten-free, depending on the brand (you must read the package label).

PT Possible reflux trigger for five percent or more people (remember, however, that any food can be a trigger).

> Some of the recipes in this book contain potential trigger foods such as sesame oil, garlic, and wine and some acids such as vinegar; for most people the amounts of these ingredients in our recipes do not cause problems. Bon appétit!

Some ingredients may be new for you and if not found in your grocery store, may be found in specialty food stores and online. Most single-ingredient and "organic" spices are actually GF, but not all. You must read the labels. We will sometimes indicate that an ingredient is "MMGF," but if you are GF, do your homework, read labels, and find your best, most-trusted brands.

Chinkiang vinegar [PT, MMGF]
  about, 90
  recipes with, 123, 152
Choy sum, 188
Cilantro, 105, 110, 112, 117, 119,
  135, 155, 169, 170–71, 172, 177,
  178, 187, 191
Cinnamon (ground), 97, 98, 205,
  208, 220
Cinnamon stick, 114–15, 207
Clams, 189
Cloves (whole and ground)
  about, 90
  recipes with, 97, 114–15, 191,
  207, 220
Collard greens, 118
Coriander (ground), 117, 129
Corn (frozen), 190
Corn, popping, 199
Cornmeal[MMGF], 100, 146, 174–75,
  175, 195
Corn on the cob, 124, 135, 159
Cornstarch[MMGF], 95, 110, 112, 119,
  172, 190, 196
Cremini mushrooms, 143, 174–75
Cucumber, 119, 129, 133, 136,
  152, 165, 210, 211
Cumin (ground), 129, 151, 180–
  81, 200–201
Cumin seeds, 117

Daikon radish, 191, 199
Daikon sprouts (kaiware), 165
Dandelions, 136, 138
Dill, 104, 125, 129, 161, 186, 217

Edamame
  about, 90
  recipe with, 132

Eggplant, 145, 200–201
Eggs, 97, 98, 102, 103, 104, 110,
  112, 119, 147, 153, 197, 198

Fennel, 148, 164, 178
Fennel seeds, 220
Fermented black beans[NGF, PT]
  about, 90
  recipe with, 157
Feta, 206
Fish. See Arctic char; Halibut;
  Salmon (smoked and roe); Sea bass
Flour (all-purpose white) [NGF], 96,
  146, 149, 174–75, 195, 205. See
  also Buckwheat flour; Garbanzo
  bean flour; Quinoa flour; Rye
  flour; Semolina flour; Whole-
  wheat flour
Frisée, 136
Fruit, seasonal, 212, 213

Garbanzo bean flour, 200–202
Garbanzo beans, 121, 129, 130
Garlic cloves [PT], 121, 189, 192, 220
Garlic-infused olive oil [PT]
  about, 90
  recipe, 220
  recipes with, 129, 138, 219
Ginger (fresh and ground), 97, 105,
  110, 112, 117, 119, 123, 150,
  155, 157, 161, 169, 170–71, 172,
  176, 177, 187, 188, 189, 191,
  196, 197, 202, 210, 220
Grapeseed oil
  about, 91
  recipes with, 96, 100, 125, 135,
  148, 156, 162, 172, 195, 200–
  201, 205
Green beans, 130, 202

Savory, 180–81

Sea bass, 187

Seaweed-mushroom stock
  recipe, 218
  recipes with, 109, 111, 116, 118, 121, 123, 124, 132, 139, 143, 154, 159, 161, 164, 179, 188, 219

Seeds. *See specific seed types*

Semolina flour^{NGF}, 182–83

Sesame oil^{PT}
  about, 92
  recipes with, 105, 112, 119, 150, 157, 170–71, 176, 179

Sesame oil, toasted
  about, 92
  recipes with, 102, 119, 137, 150, 152, 187, 196

Sesame seeds^{PT}, 132, 136, 139, 165, 219

Shallots, 178

Shaoshing wine^{PT, MMGF}. *See also* Rice wine (mijiu)
  about, 92
  recipes with, 157, 170–71, 172, 176, 188, 191

Sherry, dry^{PT}, 113, 172, 176, 188, 191

Sherry vinegar^{PT, MMGF}, 130

Shiitake mushrooms
  about, 92
  recipes with, 105, 143, 169, 170–71, 177, 188, 196, 217, 218

Shrimp, 112, 178, 185, 190, 196

Snow peas, 200–201

Soba^{NGF}, 152, 165

Somen noodles^{NGF}, 154

Soybeans, 165

Soybean sprouts, 160

Soymilk, 95, 96, 99, 100, 146, 164, 174–75, 175, 182–83, 195

Soy sauce^{MMGF}, about, 92. *See also* Tamari

Spinach, 95, 121, 139, 153

Sprouts. *See* Alfalfa sprouts; Bean sprouts; Daikon sprouts (kaiware); Radish sprouts; Soybean sprouts

Squash, butternut, 162

Squash, zucchini. *See* Zucchini

Star anise, 169, 176, 191

String beans. *See* Chinese long beans

Sugar, 169, 189. *See also* Palm (coconut) sugar

Sumac^{PT}
  about, 92
  recipes with, 121, 129

Sunflower seeds, 199

Sweet potato (preferably satsuma imo), 155, 156

Tahini^{PT}
  about, 92
  recipes with, 121, 129, 152

Tamari
  about, 92
  recipes with, 119, 123, 132, 133, 137, 139, 150, 152, 154, 155, 160, 169, 170–71, 172, 176, 179, 187, 188, 189, 191, 196, 197, 199, 202, 219

Tea, black, 197

Tea, jasmine, 207

Tempeh
  about, 92
  recipes with, 172, 174–75, 179

Thyme, 95, 111, 113, 114–15, 118, 130, 131, 134, 136, 174–75, 175, 219

Tofu, 95, 109, 112, 123, 153, 175
Tomatoes PT, 178, 200–201
Tortillas (flour) NGF, 104
Turkey (ground), 169, 184, 196, 202
Turmeric, 95, 117, 151

Vanilla, 96, 207
Vegetables, 95, 109
Vegetable stockMMGF
   about, 92
   recipe, 217
   recipes with, 111, 113, 116, 118, 120, 121, 143, 144, 151, 159, 161, 172, 186, 188, 192
Vinegar. See Balsamic vinegar; Chinkiang vinegar; Rice (wine) vinegar; Sherry vinegar

Wakame (seaweed)
   about, 92
   recipes with, 109, 133
WasabiMMGF, 154
Watercress, 120, 123
Watermelon, 206, 209
White beans, 111
White flour. See Flour (all-purpose white)
White wine PT, 111, 163
Whole-wheat flourNGF, 149

Yam, 217
Yeast (dry) NGF, 146, 149. See also Nutritional yeast

Zucchini, 185

Recommended Reading
and References

1. Koufman J, Stern J, Bauer M. *Dropping Acid: The Reflux Diet Cookbook & Cure*. The Reflux Cookbooks (2010).

2. Davis, William. *Wheat Belly*. Rodale, New York, NY (2011).

3. Lustig, Robert. *Fat Chance: Beating the Odds Against Sugar, Processed Food, Obesity, and Disease*. Plume (2013).

4. Perlmutter D, Loberg C. *Grain Brain: The Surprising Truth about Wheat, Carbs, and Sugar—Your Brain's Silent Killers*. Little, Brown and Company (2013).

5. Bittman, Mark. *A Bone to Pick*. Pam Krauss Books (2015).

6. GRAS List:
http://www.fda.gov/Food/IngredientsPackagingLabeling/FoodAdditivesIngredients/ucm091048.htm

7. Food Safety: FDA Should Strengthen Its Oversight of Food Ingredients Determined to Be Generally Recognized as Safe (GRAS). GAO-10-246: United States Government Accountability Office, February 3, 2010.

8. Koufman J. Low-Acid Diet for Recalcitrant Laryngopharyngeal Reflux: Therapeutic Benefits and Their Implications. *Ann Otol Rhinol Laryngol* 120:281-287, 2011.

9. Koufman JA. The otolaryngologic manifestations of gastroesophageal reflux disease. *Laryngoscope* 101 (Suppl. 53):1-78, 1991.

10. Belafsky PC, Postma GN, Koufman JA. Validity and reliability of the reflux symptom index (RSI). *J Voice* 16:274-7, 2002.

11. Belafsky PC, Postma GN, Koufman KA. Laryngopharyngeal reflux symptoms improve before changes in physical findings. *Laryngoscope* 111: 979-981, 2001.

12. Loughlin CJ, Koufman JA. Paroxysmal laryngospasm secondary to gastroesophageal reflux. *Laryngoscope* 106:1502-5, 1996.

13. Loughlin CJ, Koufman JA, Averill DB, et al. Acid-induced laryngospasm in a canine model. *Laryngoscope* 106:1506-9, 1996.

14. Koufman JA, Amin M, Panetti M. Prevalence of reflux in 113 consecutive patients with laryngeal and voice disorders. *Otolaryngol Head Neck Surg* 123:385-388, 2000.

15. Duke SG, Postma GN, McGuirt WF Jr, Ririe D, Averill DB, Koufman JA. Laryngospasm and diaphragmatic arrest in immature dogs after laryngeal acid exposure: a possible model for sudden infant death syndrome. *Ann Otol Rhinol Laryngol* 110:729-33, 2001.

16. Axford SE, Sharp S, Ross PE, Pearson JP, Dettmar PW, Panetti M, Koufman JA. Cell biology of laryngeal epithelial defenses in health and disease: Preliminary studies. *Ann Otol Rhinol Laryngol* 110:1099-1108, 2001.

17. Belafsky PC, Postma GN, Koufman JA. The validity and reliability of the reflux finding score (RFS). *Laryngoscope* 111:1313-17, 2001.

18. Postma GN, Tomek MS, Belafsky PC, Koufman JA. Esophageal motor function in laryngopharyngeal reflux is superior to that of classic gastroesophageal reflux disease. *Ann Otol Rhinol Laryngol* 110:1114-6, 2001.

19. Amin MR, Postma GN, Johnson P, Digges N, Koufman JA. Proton pump inhibitor resistance in the treatment of laryngopharyngeal reflux. *Otolaryngol Head Neck Surg* 125:374-8, 2001.

20. Smoak BR, Koufman JA. Effects of gum chewing on pharyngeal and esophageal pH. *Ann Otol Rhinol Laryngol* 110:1117-1119, 2001.

21. Koufman JA, Aviv JE, Casiano RR, Shaw GY. Laryngopharyngeal reflux: Position statement of the Committee on Speech, Voice, and Swallowing Disorders of the American Academy of Otolaryngology—Head and Neck Surgery. *Otolaryngol Head Neck Surg* 127:32–35, 2002.

22. Johnston N, Bulmer D, Gill GA, Panetti M, Ross PE, Pearson JP, Pignatelli M, Axford A, Dettmar PW, Koufman JA. Cell biology of laryngeal epithelial defenses in health and disease: Further studies. *Ann Otol Rhinol Laryngol* 112:481-491, 2003.

23. Johnston N, Knight J, Dettmar PW, Lively MO, Koufman J. Pepsin and carbonic anhydrase isoenzyme III as diagnostic markers for laryngopharyngeal reflux disease. *Laryngoscope* 114:2129-34, 2004.

24. Knight J, Lively MO, Johnston N, Dettmar PW, Koufman J. Sensitive pepsin immunoassay for detection of laryngopharyngeal reflux. *Laryngoscope* 115:1473-78, 2005.

25. Koufman J, Huang S, Geisberg M, Round T. A New, Inexpensive, and Non-Invasive Saliva Test for Laryngopharyngeal Reflux: Sensitivity and Specificity of a Rapid Pepsin Immunoassay (U.S. Patent 5,879,897). Presented at the Voice Foundation annual meeting, June 6, 2014.

26. Gill GA, Johnston N, Buda A, Pignatelli M, Pearson J, Dettmar PW, Koufman J. Laryngeal epithelial defenses against laryngopharyngeal reflux (LPR): Investigations of pepsin, carbonic anhydrase III, pepsin, and the inflammatory response. *Ann Otol Rhinol Laryngol* 114:913-21, 2005.

27. Johnston N, Dettmar PW, Lively MO, Koufman JA. Effect of pepsin on laryngeal stress protein (Sep70, Sep53, and Hsp70) response: Role in laryngopharyngeal reflux disease. *Ann Otol Rhinol Laryngol* 115:47-58, 2006.

28. Johnston N, Dettmar PW, Bishwokarma B, Lively MO, Koufman JA. Activity/stability of human pepsin: implications for reflux attributed laryngeal disease. *Laryngoscope* 117:1036-9, 2007.

29. Koufman JA, Block C. Differential diagnosis of paradoxical vocal fold movement. *American Journal of Speech and Hearing* 17:327-34, 2008.

30. Amin MR, Postma GN, Setzen M, Koufman JA. Transnasal esophagoscopy: A position statement from the American Broncho-Esophagological Association. *Otolaryngol Head Neck Surg* 138:411-3, 2008.

31. Koufman J, Johnston N. Potential Benefits of pH 8.8 Alkaline Drinking Water as an Adjunct in the Treatment of Reflux Disease. *Ann Otol Rhinol Laryngol* 121:431-434, 2012.

32. Koufman J. *The Chronic Cough Enigma*. Katalitix Media (2014).

33. Reavis KM, Morris CD, Gopal DV, Hunter JG, Jobe BA. Laryngopharyngeal reflux symptoms better predict the presence of esophageal adenocarcinoma than typical gastroesophageal reflux symptoms. *Ann Surg* 239:849-56, 2004.

34. Hvid-Jensen F, Pedersen L, Funch-Jensen P, Drewes AM. Proton pump inhibitor use may not prevent high-grade dysplasia and oesophageal adenocarcinoma in Barrett's oesophagus: a nationwide study of 9883 patients. *Alimentary Pharmacology and Therapeutics*, pp. 1-8, 2014.

35. Shah NH, LePendu P, Bauer-Mehren A et al. Proton pump inhibitor usage and the risk of myocardial infarction in the general population. PLoS ONE 015 Jun 10;10(6):e0124653. doi: 10.1371/journal.pone.0124653. eCollection 2015.

36. Lillemoe KD, Johnson LF, Harmon JW. Role of the components of the gastroduodenal contents in experimental acid esophagitis. *Surgery* 92:276-84, 1982.

37. Kelly EA, Samuels TL, Johnston N. Chronic pepsin exposure promotes anchorage-independent growth and migration of a hypopharyngeal squamous cell line. *Otolaryngol Head Neck Surg* 150:618-24, 2014.

38. Johnston N, Yan JC, Hoekzema CR, Samuels TL, Stoner GD, Blumin JH, Bock JM. Pepsin promotes proliferation of laryngeal and pharyngeal epithelial cells. *Laryngoscope* 122:1317-25, 2012.

39. Koufman JA, Postma GN, Whang C, Rees C, Amin M, Belafsky P, Johnson P, Connolly K, Walker F. Diagnostic laryngeal electromyography. *Otolaryngol Head Neck Surg* 124:603-606, 2001.

40. Amin MR, Koufman JA. Vagal neuropathy after upper respiratory infection: a viral etiology? *Am J Otolaryngol* 22:251-256, 2001.

41. Noar MD, Noar E. Gastroparesis associated with gastroesophageal reflux disease and corresponding reflux symptoms may be corrected by radiofrequency ablation of the cardia and esophagogastric junction. *Surg Endosc*. 22:2440-4, 2008. doi:10.1007/s00464-008-9873-4. Epub 2008 Apr 24.

42. Franciosa M, Triadafilopoulos M, Mashimo H. Stretta Radiofrequency Treatment for GERD: A Safe and Effective Modality. Gastroenterol Res Pract 2013: 783815. Published online 2013 Sep 2. doi: 10.1155/2013/783815 PMCID: PMC3775401.

43. Noar MD, Squires P, Noar E, Lee M. Long-term maintenance effect of radiofrequency energy delivery for refractory GERD: a decade later. Surg Endosc 28:2323-33, 2014. doi: 10.1007/s00464-014-3461-6. Epub 2014 Feb 22.

44. Westcott CJ, Hopkins MB, Bach KK, Postma, GN, Belafsky, PC, Koufman, JA. Fundoplication for laryngopharyngeal reflux. *American College of Surgeons* 199:23-30, 2004.

45. Pohl H, Welch HG. The role of overdiagnosis and reclassification in the marked increase of esophageal adenocarcinoma incidence. *J Natl Cancer Inst* 97:142-6, 2005.

46. Hadjivassiliou M, Grünewald RA, Chattopadhyay AK, et al. Clinical, radiological, neurophysiological, and neuropathological characteristics of gluten ataxia. *Lancet* 352:1582-5, 1998.

47. Catassi C, Elli L, Bonaz B, et al. Diagnosis of Non-Celiac Gluten Sensitivity (NCGS): The Salerno Experts' Criteria. *Nutrients* 7: 4966–77, 2015.

48. Hadjivassiliou M, Davies-Jones G, Sanders D, Grunewald R. Dietary treatment of gluten ataxia. *J Neurol Neurosurg Psychiatry*. 74:1221–24, 2003.

49. Hayeck TJ, Kong CY, Spechler SJ, et al. The prevalence of Barrett's eso-phagus in the U.S. *Dis Esophagus* 23:451-7, 2010.

50. Nestle, Marion. *Food Politics: How the Food Industry Influences Nutrition and Health.* University of California Press (2013).

51. Nestle, Marion, Bittman, Mark. *Soda Politics: Taking on Big Soda (and Winning).* Oxford University Press (2015).

52. Koufman, Jamie. The Dangers of Late Night Eating. *New York Times,* October 25, 2014.

General Index

Acid reflux. *See* Reflux
Acidic foods
    alkaline in the body fallacy, 18–19
    avoiding, 27
Acids
    FDA and harmfulness of, 25
    use of, 4–5
Acid-suppressive medications, 18
Alcohol, 27, 58
Alkaline diet, 6, 27
    goals for, 40
    maintenance phase, 41, 60–74
    rationale for, 40–41
    transition phase, 40–41, 53–59
Alkaline foods, 18–19
Alkaline water, 50–52
    benefits of, 51
    defined, 50
    drinking of, 52
    making, 52
Allergies, 13, 15
Aloe vera leaf, 50
American diet, 4
Antireflux defenses, 33–34
Antireflux medication, 17, 41–44. *See also* H2-antagonists; Proton pump inhibitors (PPIs)
    classes and brands of, 42
    use of, 41
Antireflux surgery, 45
Apple cider vinegar, 18–19
Asafoetida, 90
Asthma
    airway obstruction in, 14
    breathing IN and OUT and, 13
    misdiagnosis, 13–14
    respiratory reflux and, 15

Autoimmune diseases, 81
Avocados, 27
Bananas, 27, 50, 53–54
Barrett's esophagus
    alkaline water and, 51
    cause of, 82
    as over-diagnosed, 83
    patients, 82–84
    reflux diet modifications, 84
Beverages, 58, 73
Bicarbonate, 34
Borlaug's wheat, 76–77
Bread, 57, 77, 78
Breathing problems, 37
Brittle (Stage III), 31
Bronchitis, 14

Cancers, 15
Carbohydrate intolerance
    foot/leg cramps and, 79–80
    gluten sensitivity and, 80–81
    sugar addiction recovery and, 79
    sweet-smelling urine and, 80
Carbohydrates
    potatoes and, 27
    reducing reliance on, 79
Cheating, 73–74
Chef Philip, xiv, 63, 70–71, 87, 89
Chinkiang vinegar, 90
Chocolate, 49
Chronic cough
    as decomposition red flag, 37–38
    misdiagnosis, 14
    as neurogenic symptom, 44
The Chronic Cough Enigma (Koufman), 13, 43

in respiratory reflux assessment, 36
scores, 35–36
Reflux management, 74
Reflux Symptom Index (RSI)
defined, 3
illustrated, 3
symptoms, 9
Reflux testing, 39, 42
Remission (Stage I), 31, 32–33
Respiratory reflux
common symptoms of, 13
defined, 5, 8
diseases caused by, 10–12
misdiagnoses and, 9, 13–14
symptoms and conditions, 11
Restaurants. *See* Dining out
Rheumatoid arthritis, 81
Rice, 50

Sake, 92
Saliva, lack of, 34
Self-analysis questions, 28
Sesame oil, 92
Shaoshing wine, 92
Shiitake, 92
Sinus disease, 15
Sjogren's syndrome, 34
Snacks, in meal plan, 62, 63
Soft drinks, 6, 20, 27, 58, 78
Soy sauce, 92
Stable (Stage II), 31
Stages of reflux
defined, 30
Stage I (remission), 31, 32–33
Stage II (stable), 31
Stage III (brittle), 31
Stage IV (decompensation), 31, 32–40
Stomach acid
beverages and, 4, 58
not enough fallacy, 18

pH, 20, 51
Stretta, 45
Sugar
cutting from diet, 77
in diet, 25–26
reducing, 78
steps for quitting, 78–79
substituting, 77
types of, 77
Sugar addiction, 25–26
breaking, 26, 77, 78–79
carbohydrate intolerance and, 79
strength of, 77
Sumac, 92
Surgery, antireflux, 45
Swallowing
evaluation, 39
problems, as decomposition red flag, 37
Symptoms/conditions, reflux-related, 11

Tahini, 92
Tamari, 92
Tea, 58, 78
Tempeh, 92
Template, meal plan, 62, 64–65
Tiger-striping, 12–13, 36
Tissue inflammation, 12
Toasted sesame oil, 92
Tofu, 50
Tomatoes, 54
Trans fats, 27, 78
Transition phase
alkaline water and, 52
purpose of, 54
as trial and error, 53–59
trigger foods and, 53–57
Transnasal esophagoscopy (TNE), 39, 42, 46, 83
Trigger foods, 53–57

Index of Recipes

Acknowledgments

The authors would like to acknowledge and thank the people who inspired them and who helped refine the ideas, the manuscript, and the recipes in this book: Lisa Bromberg, Mark Flanaghan, Tom Golodik, Grace Huang, Susan Huang, Dr. Thomas Huang, Christian Janssen, Miriam Janssen, Hope Matthiessen, Dora Militaru, Tania Miller, Katie Seamans, Christopher Simpson, Latasha Taylor, Nick Tsaclas, and Katie Wilson.

About the Authors

Jamie A. Koufman, M.D., is one of the country's leading laryngologists and the Founder and Director of the Voice Institute of New York (VoiceInstitute ofNewYork.com). Dr. Koufman is also one of the world's authorities on acid reflux, and she is responsible for coining the terms *laryngopharyngeal reflux, silent reflux, airway reflux,* and *respiratory reflux*. She is Clinical Professor of Otolaryngology at the New York Eye and Ear Infirmary of Mount Sinai.

Dr. Koufman has received many honors and awards, including the Honor Award and the Distinguished Service Awards of the American Academy of Otolaryngology—Head and Neck Surgery, the Broyles-Maloney Award of the American Broncho-Esophagological Association, and the Casselberry and Newcomb Awards of the American Laryngological Association. She is a past president of the American Broncho-Esophagological Association and the New York Laryngology Society. Dr. Koufman has been listed among the Top Doctors in America every year since 1994.

Dr. Koufman is a *New York Times* best-selling author of *Dropping Acid: The Reflux Diet Cookbook & Cure* and *The Chronic Cough Enigma*.

Sonia Huang, PA-C, is a New York-based physician assistant who has been working with Dr. Koufman at the Voice Institute of New York for the past three years. Sonia's specialized medical training was in the fields of otolaryngology and gastroenterology. Sonia spent her childhood in Taiwan before moving to the United States. She graduated with a B.S. degree in neurophysiology, has a B.A. in art history from The University of Maryland, and received PA training at Long Island University. Sonia learned cooking from her grandmother, who was an accomplished chef, and many of Sonia's recipes have deep roots. Most of her contributions to *Dr. Koufman's Acid Reflux Diet* are Asian home-style cooking recipes.

Philip Gelb is a San Francisco-based vegan chef. His catering company, In the Mood for Food, has a reputation for making everything in-house and from the finest, freshest seasonal and local ingredients. His cooking classes and renowned dinner/concert series showcase Chef Philip's unique and flavorful approach to contemporary vegetarian cuisine. Visit his blog at philipgelb.blogspot.com and his website at ChefPhilipGelb.com.